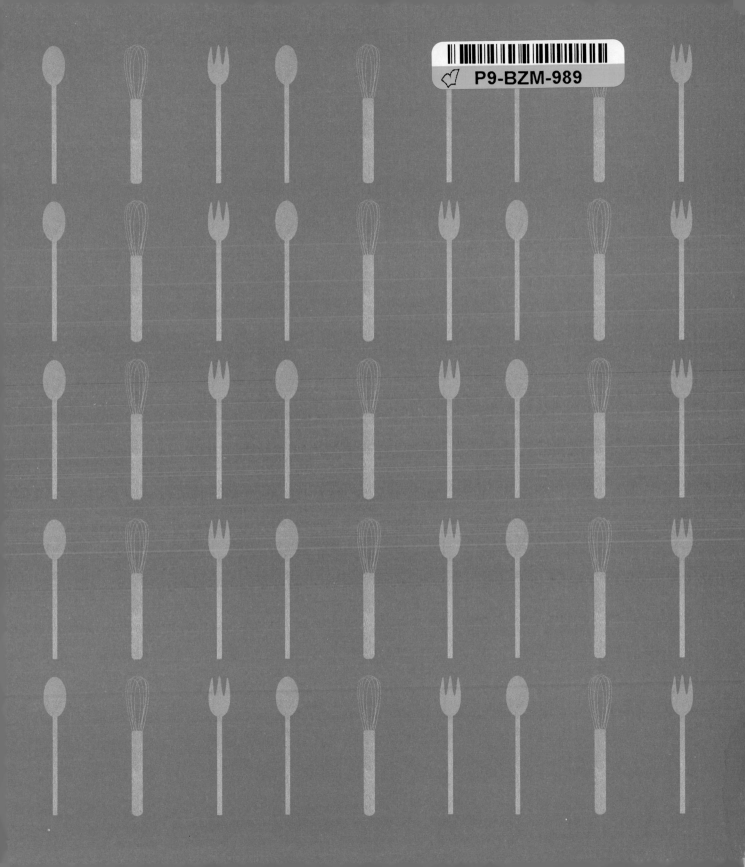

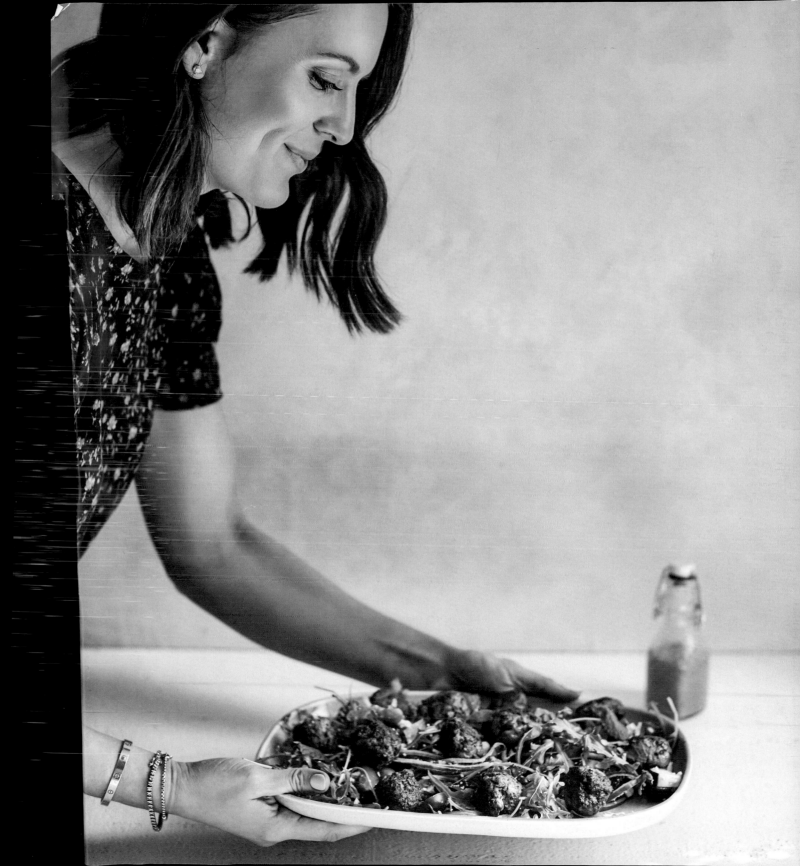

the

DEFINED DISH

the DEFINED DISH

HEALTHY AND WHOLESOME WEEKNIGHT RECIPES

ALEX SNODGRASS

Photography by **KRISTEN KILPATRICK**

Foreword by **Melissa Urban**
CO-CREATOR OF THE WHOLE30

HOUGHTON MIFFLIN HARCOURT
Boston New York 2020

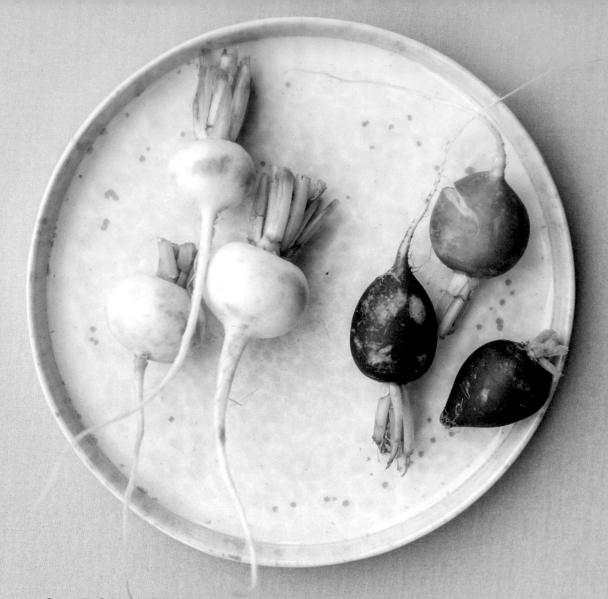

hmhbooks.com

Library of Congress Cataloging-in-Publication Data is available.

ISBN 978-0-358-00441-7 (hbk)

ISBN 978-0-358-00400-4 (ebk)

Book design by Toni Tajima

Printed in China

C&C 10 9 8 7 6 5 4 3 2 1

To the Defined Dish Community: This book would not be here without you. A huge hug to each of you for always supporting me and cheering me on every step of the way. Thank you for sharing my blog with your friends and family and for cooking my dishes. It brings me more happiness than you could ever know. I can't wait to see these recipes be made in your own homes for the ones you love most! You are so special to me, and I am so incredibly blessed to be able to share what I love with you.

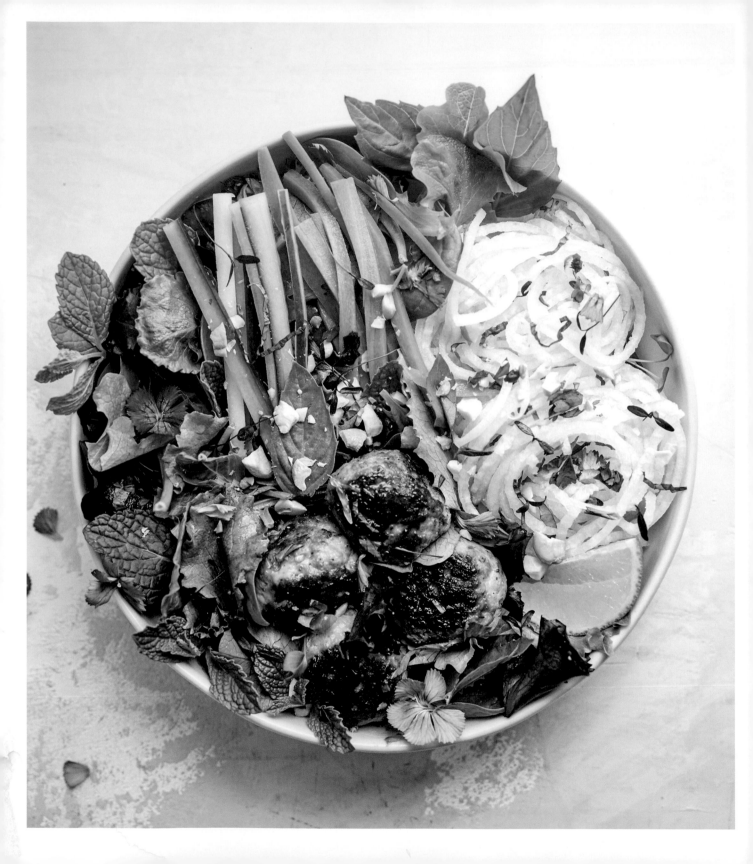

CONTENTS

ACKNOWLEDGMENTS

My sweet Sutton and Winnie: Everything I do is with you first in my heart. You make me want to wake up every day and do something great. Although I want you to stay young forever, I cannot wait until you are both old enough to cook these recipes one day. It already warms my heart thinking about it. You continue to inspire me to put my heart and soul into everything I do.

The queen, Melissa Urban: Thank you for starting the Whole30. You have changed my life in so many more ways than I could ever imagine. You not only taught me that eating clean makes me feel good, but aside from that, you taught me that taking care of myself first makes me a better human. Thank you for believing in me. I am forever grateful.

Kristen Kilpatrick: You made this book more beautiful than I could ever imagine. You are such a light to be around and I cannot imagine creating this book alongside anyone else but you. Thank you for pushing me outside of my comfort zone and making me feel beautiful in these photos. For capturing the beauty in these dishes I love so much. For spending countless hours and late nights working on this with me, and for making me laugh so hard I could pee my pants. I am lucky to call you my friend!

My funky, loving, and caring husband, Clayton: Without you, I might not stay sane doing what I do. Thank you for always talking through life's and work's obstacles. The Defined Dish wouldn't be here without you. You have encouraged me so much to pursue my dreams and have been such an important part of everything. Thank you for being my at-home Gordon Ramsay, tasting each and every one of these dishes and always providing your honest feedback. I love you more than words can say. Thank you for being my partner in life and for always lifting me up when I need you most.

Mom: Thank you for teaching me so much in the kitchen and for being a rock I can always count on. Without you, I would not be who I am today, sharing what I share and doing what I do. You've shown me how to be the strong and loving woman I am. Thank you for your undying love and support in all that I do. (Oh, and for testing like 45 of these recipes for me!)

My best friend in the world, my sister, Madison: I don't know what I'd do without you. Your friendship is one of the most important things to me in my life, and I am so grateful that God gave me a best friend through giving me a little sister. Thank you for being my ride-or-die, for testing hundreds of recipes for me, for listening to me when I need a good cry, and for pumping me up and making me feel like a rock star! I love you.

Dad: Thank you for supporting me and loving me, endlessly. Now that I am older with children, I look back on my childhood and see how much you have sacrificed for me, Madison, and Clay. Thank you for leaving your busy work day and never missing one of my sporting events or important school accomplishments, for drawing me a hot bath every night after a "long day" of being a busy kid (ha!), for waking me up at 5 a.m. for cross-country practices with a cold water and note in my car and for making me a hot breakfast every morning. You are a bada**. I am so proud to call you my Dad, and I am so grateful for the love you have shown me.

GoGo: I would have never in a million years thought I'd be so close with my mother-in-law. You have taught me so much in the kitchen, and I thank you for that. But I thank you more for teaching me the art of dedication and sacrifice. I can always rely on you for anything and I hope to do the same for my children. Thank you for all that you do for our little family, and for loving me like your own daughter. You are so special to me.

Papa: Thank you for telling every single person that you talk about to my blog. I can just see you now at lunch today telling the waiter about it, and it makes me smile. You are such a wonderful father-in-law and I am appreciative of the love and support you provide.

Clay. My big brother who always has my back, cheers me on, and helps with my technological issues in life! I love you very much.

Teri Turner: Thank you so much for being a phone call away throughout my career and the creation of this book. You have been such a wonderful mentor and friend to me. I am so grateful for your support.

Taylor: Thank you for approaching me at Whole Foods that day and asking if I needed an assistant. I really did (ha ha), and you have far exceeded my expectations. We've destroyed my kitchen far too many times together creating magic, and I look forward to many more. Thanks for being my friend, for being a part of The Defined Dish, and for being a crucial part in the creation of this book!

Justin Schwartz, my editor at Houghton, Mifflin Harcourt: Thank you for making this possible and for making my day each time you cook one of my recipes on Instagram. I am so appreciative of having an editor who loves my work and my recipes.

My dear friend, Kourtney: Thank you for recipe testing for me, even though you hate cooking! I am so glad that we went to Spain together and became sisters by choice.

Kelly and McKenzie: Thank you for taking the time out of your busy schedules and testing so many of these recipes for me. It makes me so grateful for Instagram to form friendships like yours.

Lisa Grubka at Fletcher & Company: Thank you for reaching out to me, for your encouragement, and for believing in me with such love and compassion.

Fannie, Jeanette, and Nonnie: As I wrote each of the Southern Charms recipes, I thought of you in Heaven. Thank you for showing me the art of cooking with heart and soul . . . and maybe a little bit of butter ;)

Martha, our nanny and friend: I am so thankful to have you in our lives, and to have someone that I trust so dearly help me take care of the girls so I can follow my dreams. Thank you for all that you do for our little family, for being a friend I can talk to, and for tasting all of my "Tacos y Más" recipes and providing me with your honest opinion. You always know how to spice things up in the kitchen, and I love learning from you! I hope you know how important you are to me and our family. I couldn't do all that I do with The Defined Dish without you!

Mimi: I'll never forget rolling meatballs with you in your kitchen. So many of the Italian recipes in this book are with you and Papu in my heart.

The wonderful team at Houghton Mifflin Harcourt: Thank you for your enthusiastic determination to get my first book published. I have enjoyed working with each of you so very much.

All of my blogger friends out there: Ronny, Monique, Alex, Bridget, ChinYu, Amanda, Roni, Izzah, Ashley, Serena, Kelsey, Chrissa, Monica, Michelle, Julia, Shea, Lindsay, Caroline, Carmen, Danika, Blair, Courtney, Soleil, Shannon, and Carissa (to name a few, I could go on for days!), thank you for being a friend to me. The world of social media is a weird place, but making friends like you is pretty awesome and you each inspire me so very much. Thank you for always lifting me up and supporting me.

All of my other dearest friends and family: You know who you are! I am so thankful for everything that you've done to make this book possible. From spreading the word about The Defined Dish to everyone you know and to those of you who helped test recipes from this book for me. Your support and love means the world to me. Thank you for being a big part of this journey with me.

FOREWORD

Everyone needs an Alex.

You know, that friend who can peek in your fridge, see the last of the veggies sitting in the crisper, and show you how to turn them into a delicious, hearty dinner. The one who can size up your kid's favorite meal, roll up her sleeves, and whip up an allergy-friendly, nutrient-dense version your whole family will love. The person you call when your mother-in-law/boss/love interest is coming over for dinner, and you want to wow them with flavor using ingredients you know will keep your energy, focus, and confidence high.

I've been following Alex on social media for years, and her recipes have become some of my family's favorites. A recent text from Dad read, "Made Alex's rack of lamb with mint chimichurri yesterday. It was so good, I dropped her an email thanking her for the recipe." (You can find that one on page 215; make extra chimichurri. You're welcome.) But even though I've known, and been cooking with, Alex for years, the recipes in this book still surprised and delighted me. Blueberries on steak! Curried pot roast! OKRA FRIES! Now that Alex has introduced me to this Southern favorite, I may never go back to baked sweet potato fries again.

Thanks to this Whole30 Endorsed book, you too can have Alex surprising and delighting you in your kitchen, showing you how to modify traditional dishes in a way that fits your family's health goals, recreate your favorite take-out meals with ingredients you can feel good about, and integrate your Food Freedom favorites in a way that leaves you looking and feeling your best.

Alex has brought the full force of her Texas roots and Italian heritage to these pages to inspire, nourish, and encourage your whole food, Whole30, or Food Freedom journey. Infused with grace, charm, and encouragement to cook what you love, involve the whole family, and create your own version of "balance," *The Defined Dish Wholesome Weeknights* and Alex will quickly become as beloved in your family as they are in mine.

Melissa Urban
Whole30 Co-founder and CEO

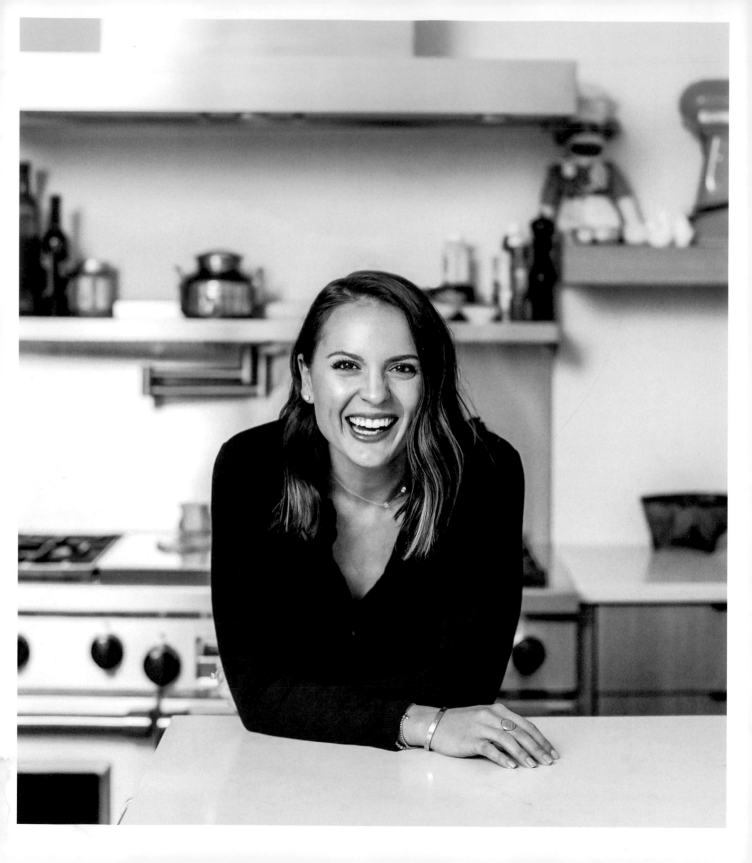

INTRODUCTION

Ever since I can remember, I have loved food. I loved gathering as a family in the kitchen each evening to help my mom with dinner. I vividly remember being a little girl and always offering up my services as her little sous chef. I would help dice tomatoes for her homemade sauce and roll out the pizza dough she made from scratch. Sitting down at the dinner table every night with my parents and siblings ranks among the fondest of my childhood memories, so to me, food = family.

If you haven't already guessed, I'm an Italian girl, which serves as an inspiration for many of my dishes, but definitely not all. Life was pretty simple in the small town where I grew up, but in the best way. Have you ever seen *Friday Night Lights*, the show about the little football-obsessed town in the middle of nowhere? That's basically Celina, Texas, in a nutshell. We didn't have easy access to all the entertainment and amenities Dallas—the closest big city—had to offer, so dinner with my loved ones was something to which I genuinely looked forward. I love my hometown and its strong sense of community. It holds an incredibly special place in my heart, and it was there that my love for cooking blossomed.

Home cooked meals were definitely the norm when I was growing up. I didn't know much else outside of Celina's only real restaurant, an infamous burger joint called Burger Fixins, and trips into the city for special occasions. I used to love loading into my dad's car on weekends to go to Dallas to shop for groceries. While my mom does most of the cooking, my dad was, and still is, the ultimate grocery shopper. We'd fill the shopping cart until it was overflowing to feed our family of five for the week. I especially loved having a say in what was going to be on the menu.

Although I loved cooking with my mom as a kid, I don't think I truly appreciated a home-cooked meal as much until my freshman year at Texas Christian University in Fort Worth. About halfway through the semester, I was beyond sick of eating not-so-tasty cafeteria food and going out to eat. I was so excited when I moved into my first apartment as a sophomore because I had my very own kitchen. Finally, I could cook dinner for myself—that's where my interest in cooking really ignited. I very quickly, and happily, became the girl who cooked for all of her friends. I absolutely loved feeding them and experimenting in the kitchen. We'd all grab a plate of whatever I had whipped up and gather around the TV to watch our favorite trashy reality TV shows. It was then that I realized I had a true passion and found myself collecting cookbooks, watching Food Network in my free time, and trying all sorts of new recipes. I was like a mad scientist discovering new techniques and flavor combinations in my kitchen every week, and I haven't stopped since.

Another love I discovered in college was my husband, Clayton! We met while both students at TCU, and you'll see me refer to him a lot throughout this book. After graduating, we moved to Austin, the capital of Texas, to start careers in politics. Each day after work, I would come home to make dinner, no matter what was going on. It was my favorite part of the day, and Clayton's too. My obsession with creating new recipes and trying new things was not slowing down, but the thought of a career in food had still never crossed my mind. Then came another life love that hadn't crossed my mind yet either—a baby.

Here we were, both young and just starting our careers, now with a baby on the way. What was next for us? I knew Clayton was my person—and Clayton knew I was his—far before I found out I was expecting. We knew we would get married eventually, so we thought, why not speed things up a bit? We did just that. We packed up our things and closed the chapter on our life together in Austin. We moved back to the Dallas–Fort Worth area to be closer to family, and not too long after our move, our sweet angel Sutton was born. It was this moment that changed my life forever in a way that I could've never imagined.

I was a new, young, stay-at-home mom, and I loved nothing more than being at home with Sutton. I was searching for work that I could do from home. I dipped my toes in the family real estate business but knew it wasn't for me. However, it was while I was working at my dad's business that I created *The Defined Dish,* a blog that I used as a creative outlet and an easy way to share my original recipes with friends and family.

Fast-forward a bit, and Clayton and I were blessed with a second beautiful daughter, Winnie. Now with two kids in tow, my life had changed dramatically, and although I was the happiest I could ever have been, I also quickly found

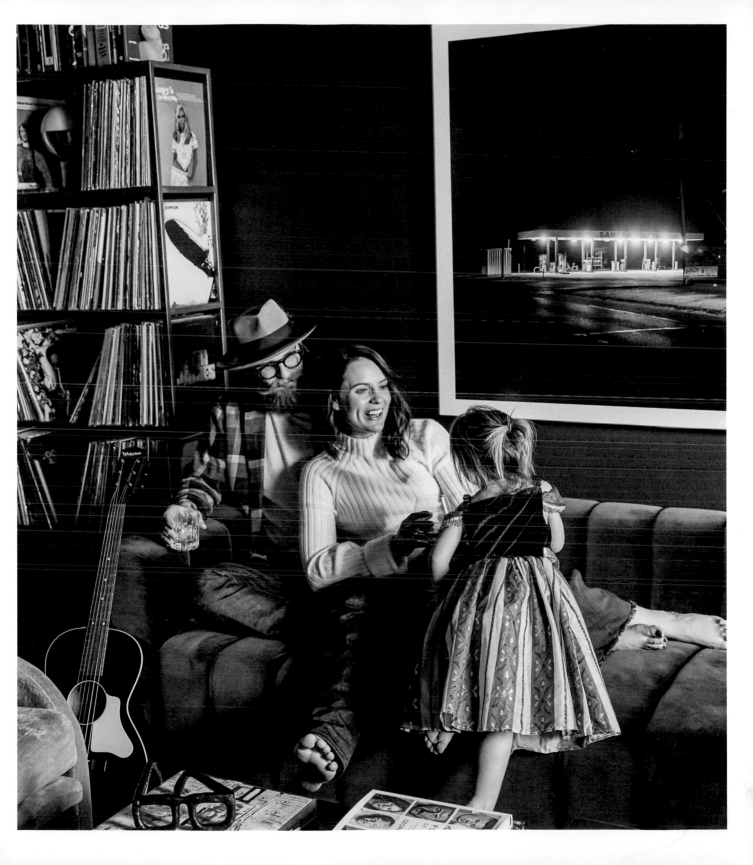

myself struggling with something I'd never experienced before—postpartum anxiety. This was all very new and scary to me, especially having grown up anxiety-free. I really didn't know how to manage it, so I was willing to try anything to help me cope with this feeling.

Enter Madison, my younger sister, who had just completed her first round of Whole30. She raved about her fantastic results and talked about how clear her mind felt. She encouraged me to do some research, and I found testimonial after testimonial about how the Whole30 helped others manage their anxiety. I knew I had to give the program a try. Thank the good Lord I did, because my life was forever changed.

The Whole30 program had incredible cognitive benefits for me. Not only did I find that the food I was consuming before was triggering my anxiety (*cough* sugar!), but over the course of 30 days, I realized the importance of self-care. As a new mom, I constantly felt buried, tending to everyone else's needs before my own. After starting the Whole30 program, I began dedicating the time I needed to my own mental and physical health. I quickly realized this didn't make me selfish but, in fact, it gave me the energy I needed to be the best mom, wife, daughter, sister, and friend I could be.

I completed my first round of Whole30 in 2015. I felt the best I had in years and knew I wanted to make this new way of approaching food a part of my everyday life. I began making easy swaps and using compliant ingredients to create delicious, wholesome meals. I posted my recipes on The Defined Dish, and I couldn't believe how many people loved them. My recipes were actually making a difference in other people's daily lives, which made me so happy. It reminded me of that feeling I would get helping my mom put a meal on the table for my family when we were kids. For me, food is more than just what fuels your body. Food brings joy into our lives, because with food we make friends, we share special moments with our loved ones, and we are reminded to count our blessings.

As far as my life after Whole30 goes, my Food Freedom is really something that ebbs and flows. Fortunately, I don't have any serious food intolerances or allergies. I choose to eat clean, real-ingredient foods simply because they make me feel good, and when I feel good, I can do great things. I love being able to indulge here and there and not feel guilty about it or punish myself. I feel strongly that my relationship with food isn't just about me—it's also about the example I'm setting for my two young girls. I hope that through my daily practices of self-love, I serve as a fantastic role model as I teach them to nourish their bodies the way that they deserve, while also supporting a healthy balance without deprivation. I never want them to live in a world where they punish themselves for eating too much pizza!

As you peruse my book, you will find a little bit of everything. These recipes are all inspired by experiences I've had in my lifetime. The Mom-bo Italiano chapter is loaded with inspiration and recipe remakes from my mom's Italian family. The Southern Charms and Tacos y Más chapters are influenced by where I was born and raised and the things I grew up eating. The rest are filled with foods I've discovered through travel, in restaurants, or via friends or family that I've adapted in my own kitchen to meet the needs of my family and our taste buds.

I am so grateful to be sharing more recipes for you to enjoy through this labor of love. I hope you enjoy cooking these recipes in your kitchens as much as I do in mine!

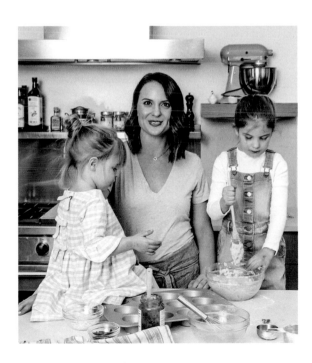

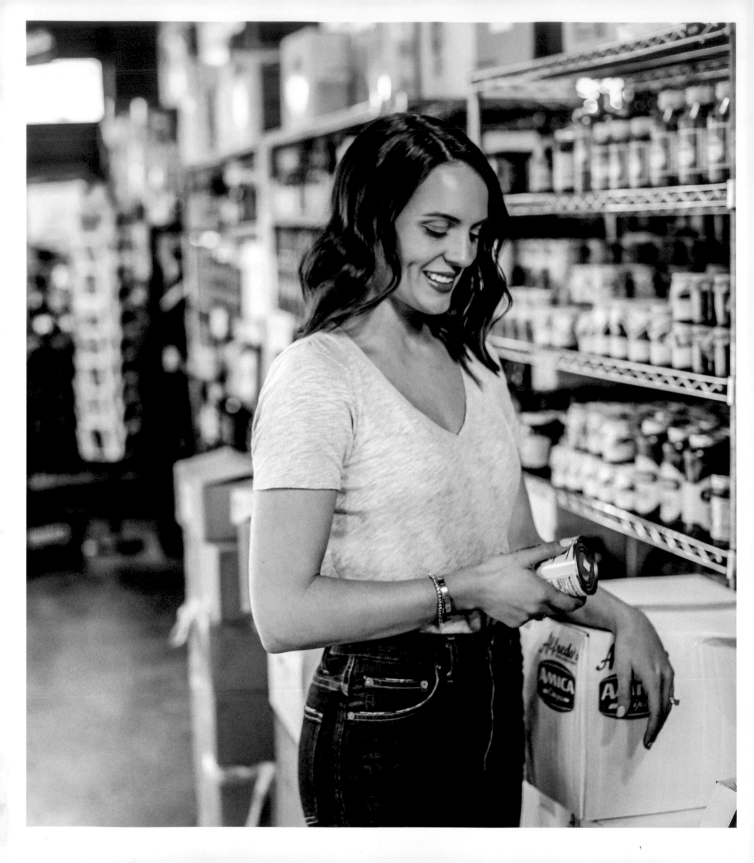

PANTRY STAPLES

Throughout this book, you'll notice there are a handful of ingredients I use quite frequently. These are ones that I always have ready in my pantry to make quick and healthy meals. Having them on-hand will be a huge help as you cook your way through this book.

GHEE Also known as clarified butter. Simply put, ghee is unsalted butter that is heated gently, causing the milk solids to separate so they can be skimmed off the top. What's left is a flavorful and Whole30-compliant cooking oil with a high smoke point. I use it just as I would regular butter—it's basically interchangeable.

COCONUT MILK In order to keep many of my dishes dairy-free, I opt for coconut milk as a substitute for things like heavy cream or cow's milk in everyday dishes. I always use unsweetened full-fat coconut milk. Be sure to check your labels! A lot of coconut milks sneak in sugar. I prefer to use Thai Kitchen brand, as I find it has a less distinctive coconut flavor, perfect for adding richness to dishes without overpowering them.

ARROWROOT STARCH Some call it arrowroot starch, some call it arrowroot flour, but it's all the same! It's a white, powdery starch extracted from the root of a tropical plant that is naturally gluten-free, grain-free, paleo, and Whole30-friendly. However, beware—some lower quality arrowroot powder blends may also contain potato starch, so be sure to check your labels. Also note that arrowroot is more similar to cornstarch than it is to flour in the way that it cooks. Like cornstarch, arrowroot is excellent for thickening soups, sauces, and gravies.

TAPIOCA STARCH Tapioca starch, also called tapioca flour, is very similar to arrowroot starch in gluten-free, Whole30 cooking; however, you'll notice

I prefer it in a few of the recipes in this book. I find that tapioca gets crisper when pan-fried, which is why I use it in recipes like my Best Grain-Free Chicken Nuggets (page 268) and Chicken-Fried Steak (page 240).

ALMOND FLOUR The finer the almond flour, the better. I use it throughout the book to add texture to recipes and sometimes to help bind. Unlike regular flour, it doesn't thicken gravies, soups, or sauces (I tend to use arrowroot starch in those types of recipes), but it is great to dredge meats in to add a crust or breading. I like to think of it as more of a replacement for breadcrumbs and panko.

COCONUT AMINOS Derived from the nectar of a coconut, coconut aminos are great for replacing traditional soy sauce in Whole30 and paleo cooking. They lend a salty, sweet flavor to dishes that is absolutely delicious; however, I never use them in my Asian-inspired dishes without the addition of Red Boat fish sauce (see below) when trying to replicate the flavor of soy sauce. Without the pairing of the fish sauce, the coconut aminos can be a little too sweet. You can find coconut aminos at most grocery stores in the Asian aisle.

RED BOAT FISH SAUCE This is one of the few ingredients in the world that bring an immediate, show-stopping umami flavor to a dish. If you've never used it before, you're going to be intimidated by its pungent smell the first time you open the bottle, but (just like anchovies) it's a secret weapon in the kitchen for big, bold, fantastic flavor. It provides a salty, briny, and slightly sweet flavor that is great in stir-fries, marinades, salad dressings, and more. I only use Red Boat brand, as most other fish sauces have added sugar.

NOURISH.
NOT PUNISH.

My Secret to Finding Balance

The million-dollar question we hear everyone asking is: "How do you find balance?" Unfortunately, I don't have the million-dollar answer. If I did, I'd be a billionaire. Just like Melissa Hartwig Urban preaches in her book *Whole30's Food Freedom Forever,* there is no one-size-fits-all diet, and balance looks different for everyone. However, I do have a philosophy that works for me and keeps me on track so that I can maintain a healthy mindset and healthy relationship with food: I "Nourish. Not Punish."

We've all had those times, whether it be a vacation, the holiday season, a big weekend of celebrating, or just a stressful week where we get off track. I am the type of person that when I go on vacation, I'm down to treat myself and indulge a bit. Bring on the tacos, margaritas, and quesadillas (if I'm in Mexico, ha-ha)! Of course, traveling and indulging on occasion leads to bloating, but you know what? It's okay to be bloated sometimes.

Here is the thing though: so many of us have gotten in this mindset that when we have a rendezvous with overindulging, we come home and restrict ourselves. Perhaps you do a juice cleanse all week, or eat tiny salads that satisfy you for what, maybe half an hour? Or perhaps you eat as little as possible and overexercise to counterbalance, punishing yourself for splurging a bit. Thanks to the Whole30 and its new mindset, I have put an end to that kind of behavior. It doesn't do any of us any good.

For me (and many), this punishment mentality leads to yo-yo dieting, and it's pretty obvious as to why. By the end of my week of restriction, I'm just going to be *really, really* hungry, plus exhausted and stressed from thinking about how hungry I've been all week. And guess what's going to happen come Friday night? I'll go out and eat all of the unhealthy things I've been missing. Bring on the fried chicken, pizza, and pasta—this girl needs some food! And so, the vicious cycle continues, and I'm stuck spending the weekends overindulging and the weekdays depriving myself.

It doesn't have to be this way. I know because I've put an end to that, and it feels so good to say "see you later" to that sort of punishment. So what exactly is it that I do when I enjoy myself a little too much? I get home and put my best foot forward. It's like reverse psychology for your body and mind. I give myself much love and nourishment with clean-ingredient, real-food meals that make me feel good, and guess what? By the end of the week, I feel like I'm back to my old self. The inflammation is gone (or at least getting close), and I feel mentally in control. It's quite liberating once you've gotten in the swing of things. It makes you realize that YOU are the only one who has the power to control your health and well-being. YOU are the one who can find a balance for yourself by setting daily intentions to nourish your body. And if you step way out of bounds for a few days or a week . . . it will all be okay. You're too beautiful a human being to punish yourself. I promise.

Each day that I have on this earth is such a blessing. I've got two beautiful young girls who look up to me, and I can only do my best each day to set a good example for them and encourage them to have a healthy relationship with food and their bodies. This book is filled with recipes that aren't just made with love, they are made with real, clean ingredients so that you can fuel your body, nourish it every week the way that it deserves, and not feel hungry or deprived. I hope you remember this love note from me to you next time you are feeling guilty after overindulging. It's all going to be okay. Let's just keep it clean this week.

So, how do you find balance? Who knows if the perfect balance is ever really attainable, but we can all do our best, and that is enough.

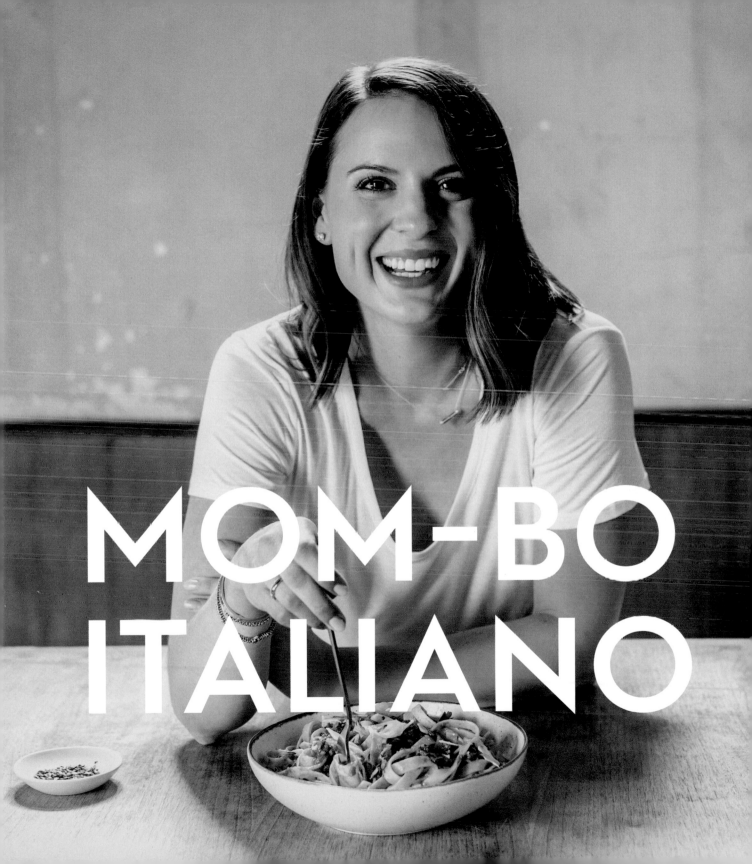

MOM-BO ITALIANO

SERVES 6

→ GLUTEN-FREE

→ DAIRY-FREE

→ PALEO

→ WHOLE30

→ GRAIN-FREE

Total time: 45 MINUTES

FOR THE MARINARA

2 tablespoons extra virgin olive oil

½ cup finely diced yellow onion (¼ medium)

2 garlic cloves, minced

½ teaspoon crushed red pepper flakes (optional)

1 tablespoon tomato paste

1 (28-ounce) can whole peeled tomatoes (I like San Marzano)

1 (15-ounce) can tomato sauce

¼ cup low-sodium beef broth

¼ cup chopped fresh flat-leaf parsley leaves

¼ cup fresh basil leaves, thinly sliced into ribbons, plus more for topping

1 teaspoon dried oregano

1 teaspoon kosher salt

½ teaspoon ground black pepper

FOR THE MEATBALLS
(on following page)

PERFECT WHOLE30 ITALIAN MEATBALLS in MARINARA SAUCE

One of my fondest memories from childhood is sitting around the kitchen table rolling meatballs with my mom while the smell of homemade marinara simmering on the stovetop filled the house. To this day, when I visit my parents and my mother is making meatballs for dinner, I feel five years old again. I've taken my mom's classic recipe and given it a grain-free, Whole30 twist. It still hits the spot, and I still get to enjoy rolling meatballs with my little girls just like I did with Mom.

MAKE THE MARINARA In a large pot over medium heat, heat the olive oil. Add the onion, garlic, and red pepper flakes (if using) and cook, stirring, until the onion is tender, about 5 minutes. Add the tomato paste and cook to soften it a bit, 1 to 2 minutes more.

Add the tomatoes and use a spoon to break them up slightly. They will continue to fall apart while cooking, so they don't have to be perfect! Stir in the tomato sauce, broth, parsley, basil, oregano, salt, and pepper. Bring to a boil, reduce to a low simmer, and cook, uncovered and stirring occasionally, while you prepare the meatballs, for about 20 minutes.

MAKE THE MEATBALLS Line a large plate with parchment paper and set aside. In a large bowl, combine the beef, almond flour, eggs, cassava flour, parsley, garlic, salt, pepper, and oregano. Using your hands, mix the meat until it is well combined. Form the mixture into 1½-inch balls (1½-tablespoon/#40 scoop) and place them on the parchment-lined plate.

In a large skillet over medium-high heat, heat the oil. Working in batches so as not to overcrowd the pan, fry the meatballs until

{ continued }

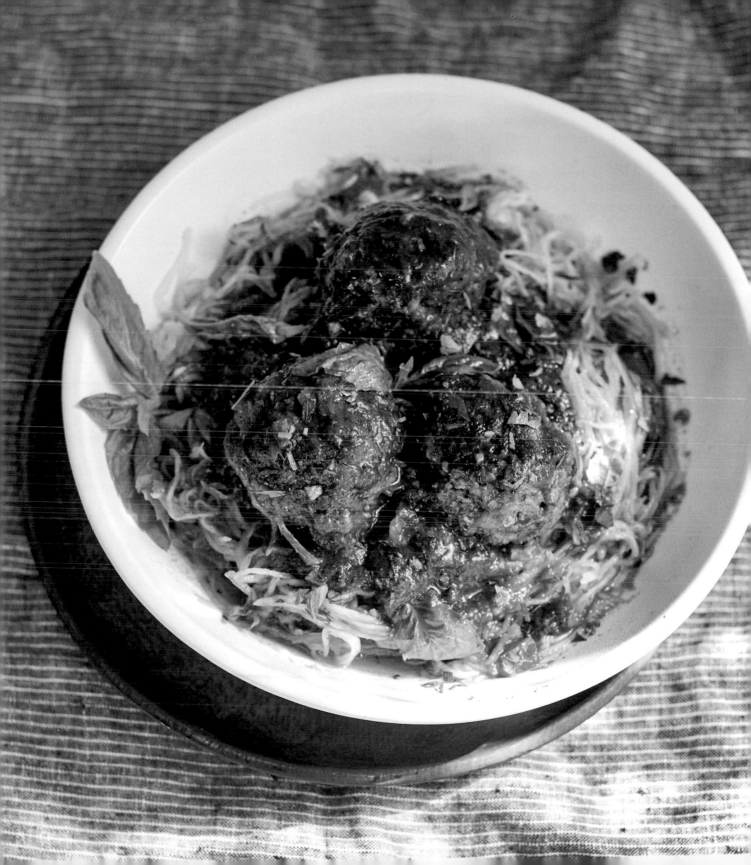

FOR THE MEATBALLS

- 2 pounds ground beef (80 percent lean)
- ½ cup almond flour
- 2 large eggs, beaten
- 1 tablespoon cassava flour
- 1 tablespoon chopped fresh flat-leaf parsley leaves
- 2 garlic cloves, minced
- 1 teaspoon kosher salt
- ½ teaspoon ground black pepper
- ½ teaspoon dried oregano
- 2 tablespoons extra virgin olive oil

Your favorite cooked pasta, zucchini noodles, or spaghetti squash (page 284), for serving (optional)

golden brown, 3 to 4 minutes per side. They don't have to be cooked through; they will continue to cook in the sauce.

Transfer the browned meatballs to the pot with the marinara sauce and simmer until the meatballs are fully cooked, 15 to 20 minutes. I suggest testing a meatball for doneness by cutting open to ensure they are cooked through, or no longer pink. When the meatballs are done, taste the sauce and season with more salt and pepper, if desired.

If desired, serve the meatballs with the sauce over your favorite pasta, zucchini noodles, or spaghetti squash. Top with remaining fresh basil, if desired.

SKILLET CHICKEN PICCATA

SERVES 4

→ GLUTEN-FREE

→ DAIRY-FREE

→ PALEO

→ WHOLE30

→ GRAIN-FREE

Total time: 40 MINUTES

Growing up, my favorite dish that my mom made was her baked lemon chicken. I crave this dish on the reg, so I still have her make it for me when I go home. I very much look forward to these chicken cutlets baked in a thick, rich, buttery lemon sauce. This is my version, which I make in a skillet for even easier weeknight prep. I also use clean, Whole30-compliant ingredients, but don't worry, it's still just as decadent and comforting as the original.

Season the chicken cutlets on both sides with the salt and pepper and set aside.

Pour the arrowroot onto a large plate or a wide bowl. Lightly dredge each individual cutlet in the arrowroot until evenly coated, then shake off any excess. Place the dredged cutlets on a clean plate and continue until all are complete.

In a large skillet over medium-high heat, heat the oil. Working in batches so as to not overcrowd the skillet, carefully add the cutlets and cook until golden brown on both sides, 3 to 4 minutes

{ continued }

- 2 pounds skinless, boneless chicken cutlets (see Note)
- 1 teaspoon kosher salt
- ½ teaspoon freshly ground black pepper
- ¼ cup arrowroot starch
- 2 tablespoons extra virgin olive oil, plus more as needed
- 1 tablespoon ghee
- 3 garlic cloves, minced
- 2 heaping tablespoons capers, drained and rinsed, plus more for serving
- 1 cup low-sodium chicken broth
- 2 tablespoons fresh lemon juice (1 lemon), plus lemon slices for garnish (optional)
- 1 tablespoon chopped fresh flat-leaf parsley leaves, for serving

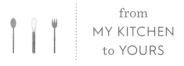

from MY KITCHEN to YOURS

A chicken cutlet is a chicken breast that has been butterflied so it opens like a book. You can either do this yourself, or purchase it already done. Once you have opened your chicken into "cutlets," finish the cut through the center so that they are divided in half lengthwise and no longer attached to each other. You should be left with two separate, thin pieces of chicken.

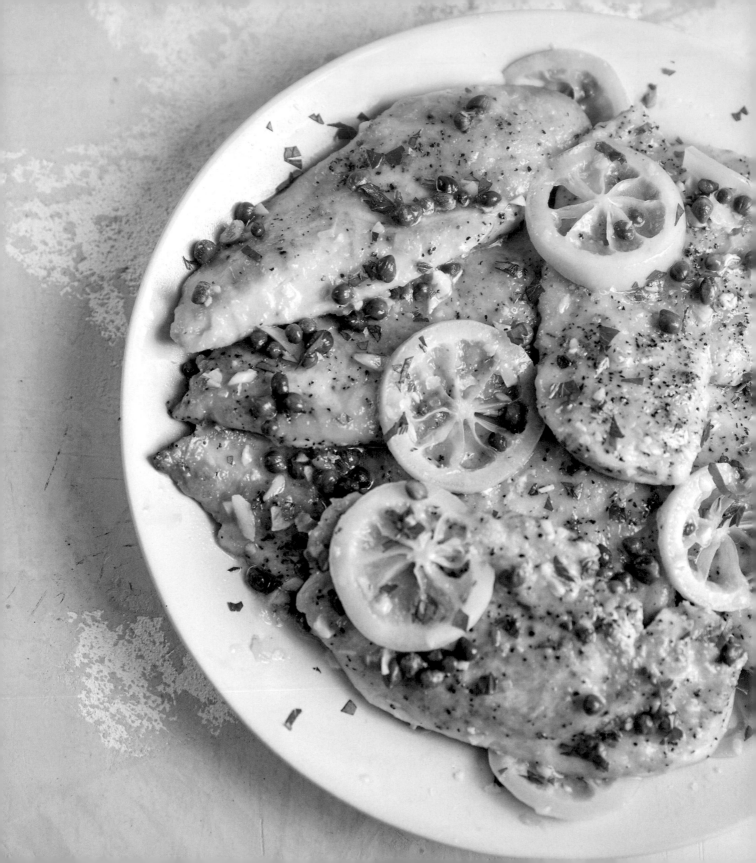

per side. The chicken does not need to be completely cooked through, just golden brown. Transfer to a parchment-lined plate. Repeat with the remaining chicken, adding more oil to the pan if necessary.

Reduce the heat to low, add the ghee to the skillet, and swirl to evenly coat the bottom of the pan. Add the garlic and cook until fragrant, stirring to prevent burning, about 30 seconds. Stir in the capers, chicken broth, and lemon juice. Increase the heat to a simmer. Nestle the chicken into the sauce and cook, uncovered and stirring occasionally, until the sauce has thickened and the chicken is tender, about 15 minutes. Taste and adjust the seasoning with salt and pepper, if desired. Garnish with the parsley and fresh lemon slices, if desired, and serve.

SERVES 4

→ GLUTEN-FREE

→ DAIRY-FREE

→ PALEO IF MODIFIED

→ WHOLE30 IF MODIFIED

→ GRAIN-FREE

Total time: 60 MINUTES

CHICKEN SALTIMBOCCA ROLL-UPS

4 (6-ounce) boneless, skinless chicken breasts

8 slices prosciutto

2 tablespoons Dijon mustard

½ teaspoon kosher salt

½ teaspoon freshly ground black pepper

1 bunch asparagus, woody ends trimmed

8 fresh sage leaves

¼ cup arrowroot starch

¼ cup plus 1 tablespoon extra virgin olive oil

2 garlic cloves, minced

½ cup low-sodium chicken broth

¼ cup dry white wine (sub more chicken broth for Whole30, paleo)

2 tablespoons fresh lemon juice (1 lemon)

Saltimbocca is an Italian dish made of veal or chicken that's wrapped with prosciutto and sage and draped with a rich wine sauce. It's a little salty, a little rustic, and absolutely scrumptious. I've adjusted the classic recipe to make these delicious Chicken Saltimbocca Roll-Ups, which are rolled with a little Dijon and asparagus, seared, and finished off in the oven in a delicious pan sauce for a complete weeknight meal in a cute little bundle of foodie love. There are quite a few steps to make this dish; however, the ingredients are simple and the end result is worth it. This is one the whole family will devour.

Preheat the oven to 400°F.

Halve the breasts into cutlets or slice them lengthwise through their equators. To do this, put one chicken breast on a cutting board and place your non-dominant hand flat on top of it. Hold a sharp knife with a smooth blade in your dominant hand. Keeping the blade parallel to the cutting board, make an even, horizontal slice through the breast, starting from the thick end and working your way toward the thin end. Repeat with the remaining chicken breasts. You should have 8 cutlets.

Place a sheet of parchment paper on top of the cutlets and use a meat mallet or the bottom of a skillet to pound each cutlet until it is an even ¼ inch thick. Transfer the cutlets to a plate and set aside.

On a (cleaned) cutting board, arrange the prosciutto slices next to one another and layer one chicken cutlet on top of

{ continued }

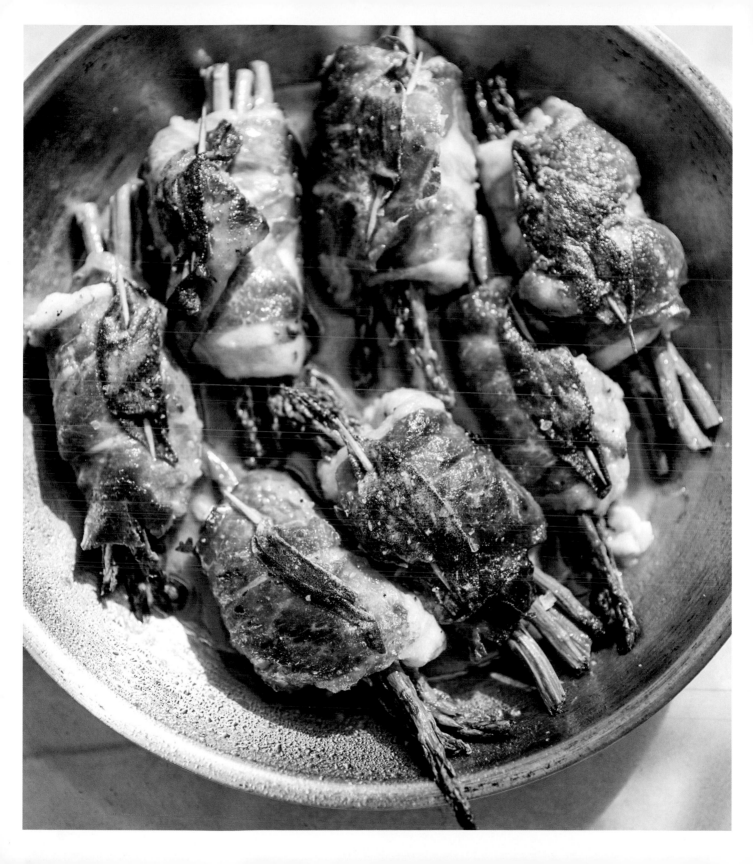

each slice. Using a brush or the back of a spoon, spread a thin layer of the mustard on the top of each cutlet. Lightly season with salt and pepper. Lay 3 stalks of asparagus at the bottom, perpendicular to the cutlet . Use the prosciutto to gently roll the chicken and asparagus into little bundles, flipping the rolls over so the seam side faces up. Place a sage leaf on top of the seam and thread a toothpick through it like a safety pin to fasten the chicken roll together and secure the sage leaf on top.

Pour the arrowroot onto a large plate or wide bowl. Gently roll each roll-up in the arrowroot to lightly dust, shaking off the excess. Set each roll-up aside on a plate and continue until all the roll-ups are coated.

In a large oven-safe skillet over medium-high heat, heat ¼ cup of the olive oil. Place the roll-ups in the skillet sage-side down and cook until golden brown and crispy, 3 to 4 minutes. You may need to work in two batches so as not to overcrowd the pan. Flip the bundles over and crisp the other side, cooking for an additional 3 to 4 minutes. Transfer the browned roll-ups to a clean plate and continue until all the roll-ups are browned.

Wipe the skillet dry and heat the remaining 1 tablespoon of olive oil over medium heat. Add the garlic and cook until fragrant, being careful not to burn it, for about 1 minute. Add the chicken broth, white wine (if using), and lemon juice and bring the mixture to a simmer. Nestle the bundles into the sauce, sage-side up, then transfer the pan to the oven, uncovered. Bake until the chicken is cooked through and the asparagus is tender, 10 to 12 minutes.

To serve, remove the toothpicks and spoon the pan sauce over the roll-ups.

STROZZAPRETI PASTA *with* SPINACH, MUSHROOMS, *and* TOASTED PINE NUTS

SERVES 4

→ GLUTEN-FREE IF MODIFIED

Total time: 35 MINUTES

There is this Italian restaurant with many locations across the United States, North Italia, that I really love. Once I tried their strozzapreti pasta dish, it's hard for me to order anything else on the menu. It's got a creamy roasted mushroom sauce that you just can't stop eating and I knew I had to re-create a lightened-up version in my own kitchen—which is just what I have done here. This is one of my go-to dishes when I am having a major pasta craving. I love how simple the recipe is, yet it always knocks me off my feet!

Heat a large, high-sided skillet over medium heat. Add the pine nuts and toast, stirring, until golden brown, 2 to 3 minutes. Transfer the nuts to a bowl and set aside. Set aside the skillet for later.

Bring a large pot of water to a boil and add the dried pasta. Cook according to the package instructions until al dente. Reserve 2 cups of the pasta water and drain the rest of the pasta in a colander. Set aside.

Reheat the large skillet over medium heat. Add the olive oil, garlic, shallot, and red pepper flakes and cook, stirring, until the shallot is tender, about 3 minutes. Add the sliced mushrooms and the broth and increase the heat to medium-high. Cook, stirring, until the mushrooms are tender, about 3 minutes. Add the cooked pasta and the Parmesan and stir to combine. Stir in

{ continued }

¼ cup pine nuts

1 pound dried strozzapreti or casarecce pasta (or brown rice pasta if gluten-free)

2 tablespoons extra virgin olive oil

3 garlic cloves, minced

¼ cup finely diced shallot (1 large)

½ teaspoon crushed red pepper flakes

3 cups thinly sliced baby bella mushrooms (8 to 10 mushrooms)

½ cup low-sodium chicken broth or vegetable broth

¾ cup freshly grated Parmesan cheese, plus more for serving

¼ cup fresh lemon juice (2 lemons)

4 cups packed baby spinach

Kosher salt and freshly ground black pepper

Chopped fresh flat-leaf parsley leaves, for serving

Lemon wedges, for serving

⅔ cup of the reserved pasta water and cook until the pasta water reduces and the sauce is light and creamy, about 3 minutes. Add the lemon juice and stir in the spinach, 2 cups at a time until it is just wilted, about 2 more minutes. Sprinkle in the toasted pine nuts.

If your pasta seems dry, ladle in the remaining reserved pasta water about a ¼ cup at a time until it rehydrates and becomes creamy. Season with salt and pepper to taste. To serve, top with Parmesan, chopped parsley, and a wedge of lemon. Enjoy!

from
MY KITCHEN
to YOURS

This is a great meatless meal, but you can add shredded chicken (page 279) if you want some extra protein. I also love serving this alongside grilled hot Italian sausages.

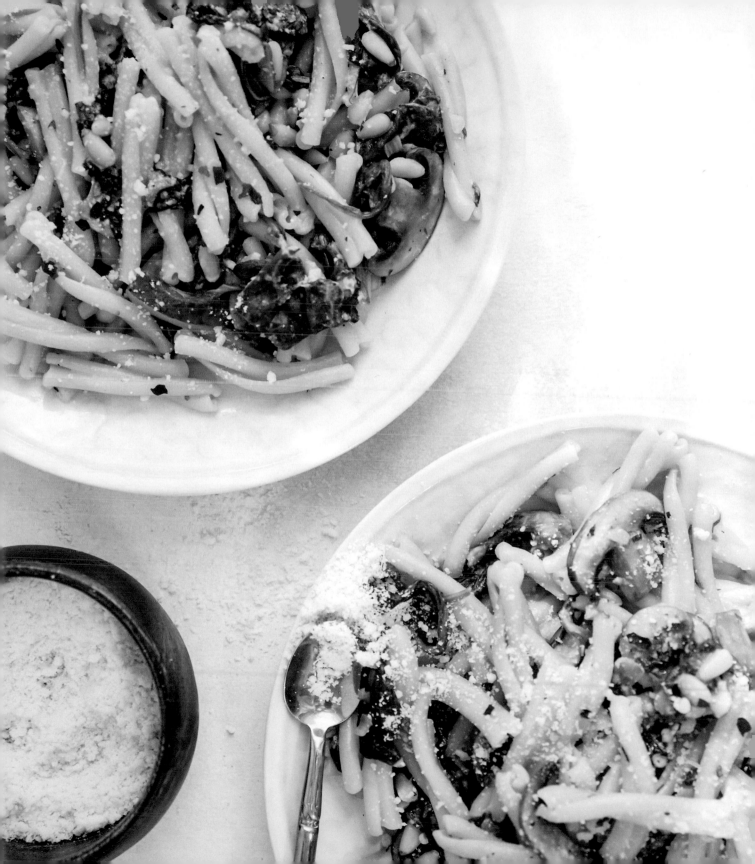

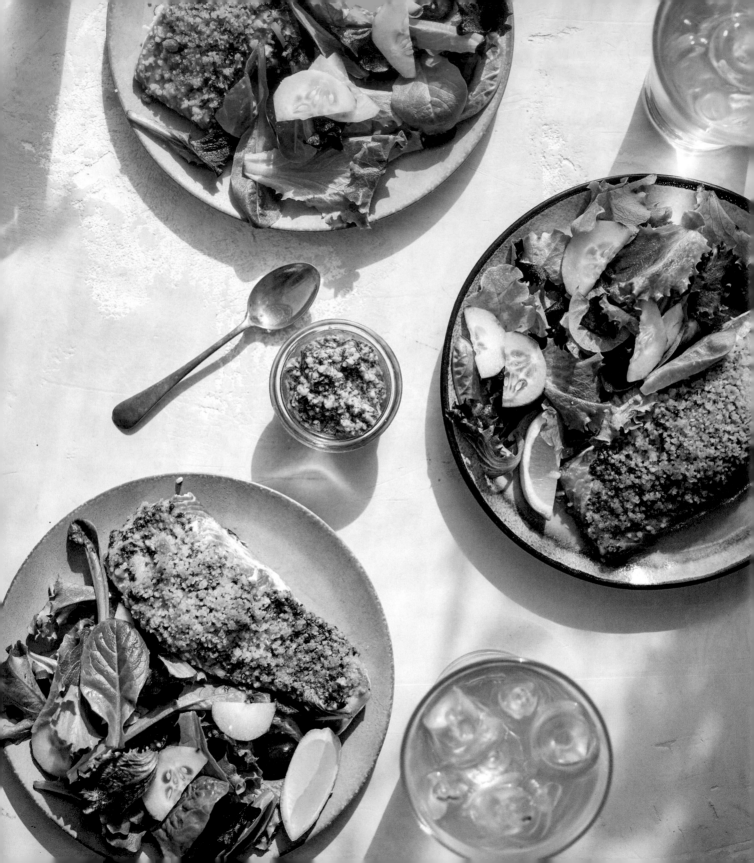

SALMON MILANO *with* LEMON-BASIL PESTO

SERVES 4
→ GLUTEN-FREE
→ DAIRY-FREE
→ PALEO IF MODIFIED
→ WHOLE30 IF MODIFIED
→ GRAIN-FREE IF MODIFIED
Total time: 35 MINUTES

This lemon-basil pesto is one of those sauces that I always want in my back pocket at all times. In fact, I always make a double batch and freeze it in small baby food containers so that I can elevate my everyday dishes in no time! This easy salmon dish is super simple to make and a crowd-pleasing weeknight meal in my home. I love the subtle crunch of the breadcrumbs on top, but you can certainly leave them out if you want to keep things Whole30.

Preheat the oven to 375°F and line a large baking sheet with parchment paper.

MAKE THE PESTO In a blender or food processor, combine the basil, olive oil, cashews, garlic, pine nuts, and lemon juice and blend until smooth. Taste and add salt and pepper to your taste. Blend once more and set aside.

MAKE THE SALMON If you're making the panko crust, toss together the breadcrumbs with the olive oil in a medium bowl until well combined. Set aside.

Arrange the salmon on the prepared baking sheet and spread 3 to 4 tablespoons of the pesto over the top of each fillet. Sprinkle evenly with the breadcrumbs, if using, and add a pinch each of salt and pepper. Bake for 15 to 20 minutes, until the salmon flakes easily with a fork.

FOR THE LEMON-BASIL PESTO

- 2 cups packed fresh basil leaves
- ½ cup extra virgin olive oil
- ⅓ cup roasted, salted cashews
- 3 garlic cloves
- 2 tablespoons pine nuts
- 2 tablespoons fresh lemon juice (1 lemon)
  Kosher salt and freshly ground black pepper

FOR THE SALMON

- ¼ cup gluten-free panko breadcrumbs (optional; I use Ian's brand) (omit for Whole30, paleo, grain-free)
- 1 tablespoon extra virgin olive oil (optional)
- 4 (6- to 8-ounce) salmon fillets
  Kosher salt and freshly ground black pepper

SERVES 4

→ GLUTEN-FREE

→ DAIRY-FREE IF MODIFIED

→ PALEO IF MODIFIED

→ WHOLE30 IF MODIFIED

→ GRAIN-FREE IF MODIFIED

Total time: 45 MINUTES

WEEKNIGHT LAMB BOLOGNESE

2 ounces sliced pancetta, finely diced

¾ cup finely diced carrot (1 medium)

¾ cup finely diced yellow onion (½ medium)

3 garlic cloves, minced

¼ teaspoon crushed red pepper flakes

1½ pounds ground lamb

½ teaspoon kosher salt

½ teaspoon freshly ground black pepper, or more to taste

1 cup dry red wine (use low-sodium beef broth for Whole30, paleo)

2 bay leaves

1 teaspoon dried thyme

3½ cups store-bought marinara sauce (I like Rao's)

½ cup whole milk (omit for Whole30, paleo, dairy-free)

1 pound fettuccine pasta (I use Cappello's grain-free pasta), cooked according to the package instructions, or spaghetti squash (page 284) for Whole30, paleo

½ cup freshly shaved Parmesan cheese (omit for Whole30, paleo, dairy-free), for serving

2 tablespoons chopped fresh flat-leaf parsley, for serving

Growing up, my mom would make a fantastic, traditional Bolognese sauce using a trio of ground meats (beef, veal, and pork) and let it simmer for hours. To this day, it is still one of my favorite things that she makes. I love making my mom's sauce on special occasions, but for weeknights I use this version instead. It takes much less time to prepare (only 45 minutes instead of hours), and I use lamb instead of all three meats, which adds rich, hearty flavor that's oh-so-satisfying.

In a high-sided saucepan or saucepot over medium heat, cook the pancetta, tossing occasionally, until just browned, 2 to 3 minutes. (It doesn't need to be fully cooked or crispy—it will continue to cook as you add the other ingredients.) Add the carrot, onion, garlic, and red pepper flakes and increase the heat to medium-high. Cook until the veggies are slightly tender, 3 to 4 more minutes. Add the lamb, salt, and black pepper. Cook, breaking up the meat with the back of a spoon, until the lamb is brown and cooked through or no longer pink, 5 to 7 minutes. Drain off any excess fat.

Stir in the red wine, bay leaves, and thyme and bring to a rapid simmer. Cook, stirring, until the wine reduces and there is only a small amount of liquid left in the pot, 3 to 5 minutes. Add the marinara sauce and bring to a boil. Reduce the heat to a light simmer and continue cooking, stirring often, until the sauce has thickened, 15 to 20 minutes.

{ continued }

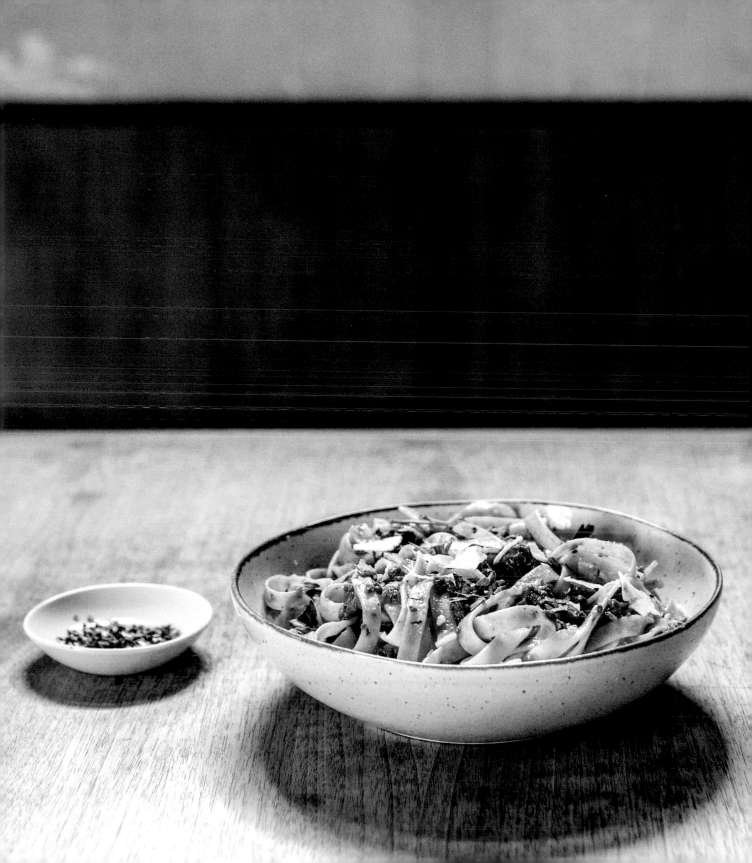

Discard the bay leaves and stir in the milk, if using. Let the sauce continue to simmer, stirring occasionally, for 10 more minutes.

Serve the Bolognese spooned over the cooked pasta or spaghetti squash and top with the Parmesan cheese and chopped parsley, if desired.

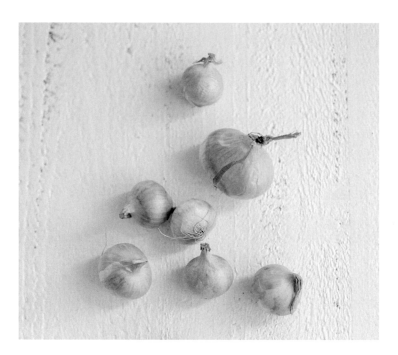

from
MY KITCHEN
to YOURS

To keep this recipe dairy-free, omit the milk and Parmesan cheese.

SHEET PAN HALIBUT *with* ITALIAN SALSA VERDE *and* ASPARAGUS

SERVES 4

→ GLUTEN-FREE

→ DAIRY-FREE

→ PALEO

→ WHOLE30

→ GRAIN-FREE

Total time: 30 MINUTES

Here is one of those super-impressive meals that also happens to take very little effort. Why? Because halibut is one of the best fish ever! Seriously. It has a light, clean flavor and buttery, flaky texture, so it doesn't take much for it to be delicious. I simply roast mine with olive oil, salt, and pepper, then top it with a bright Italian salsa verde, or "green sauce." If you've never had a salsa verde, think of it as essentially an Italian-style chimichurri, with olive oil, red wine vinegar, garlic, and tons of fresh parsley. It's absolutely delicious on pretty much anything, but I especially love it drizzled over the top of the halibut.

Preheat the oven to 400°F and line a large baking sheet with parchment paper.

MAKE THE SALSA VERDE In a food processor or blender, combine the parsley, olive oil, anchovies, capers, red wine vinegar, lemon zest, lemon juice, garlic, and red pepper flakes. Pulse until the parsley is well chopped but not pureed, scraping down the sides as needed. Set aside.

MAKE THE FISH Place the asparagus on a large sheet pan. Drizzle with 1 tablespoon of the olive oil and season with ½ teaspoon of the salt and ¼ teaspoon of the pepper. Toss to coat the asparagus and spread it over the sheet pan in a single even layer. Bake for

{ continued }

FOR THE ITALIAN SALSA VERDE

- 1 cup packed fresh flat-leaf parsley leaves
- ½ cup extra virgin olive oil
- 2 anchovy fillets
- 1 tablespoon capers, drained
- 1 tablespoon red wine vinegar
  Grated zest of 1 lemon
- 1 tablespoon fresh lemon juice (½ lemon)
- 2 garlic cloves
- ¼ teaspoon crushed red pepper flakes

FOR THE HALIBUT

- 1 bunch of asparagus, woody ends trimmed
- 3 tablespoons extra virgin olive oil
- 4 (5-ounce) halibut fillets (see Note)
- 1 teaspoon kosher salt
- ½ teaspoon freshly ground black pepper
- 1 lemon, cut into wedges, for serving

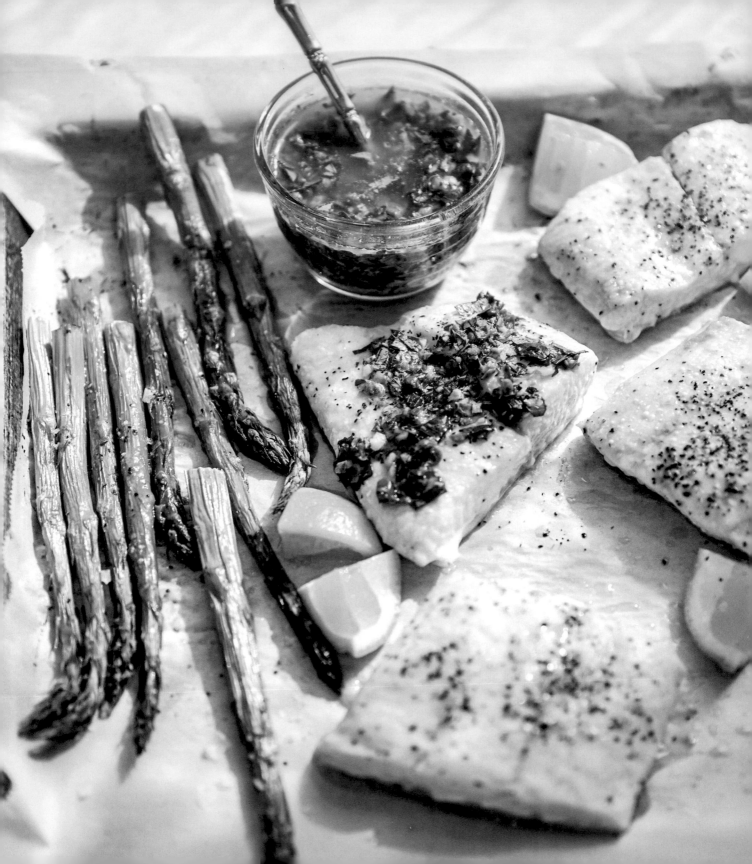

7 minutes, just to partially cook the asparagus. Remove the baking sheet from the oven and push the asparagus to the sides of the pan to make room for the fish in the center.

Place the halibut fillets on the empty side of the baking sheet. Drizzle the fillets with the remaining 2 tablespoons olive oil and season the tops with the remaining ½ teaspoon salt and ¼ teaspoon pepper. Return the pan to the oven and bake until the halibut flakes easily with a fork and the asparagus is tender, 12 to 14 minutes. Serve hot with the Italian salsa verde and lemon wedges.

from
MY KITCHEN
to YOURS

You could make this recipe with any white flaky fish such as cod, fluke, or striped bass.

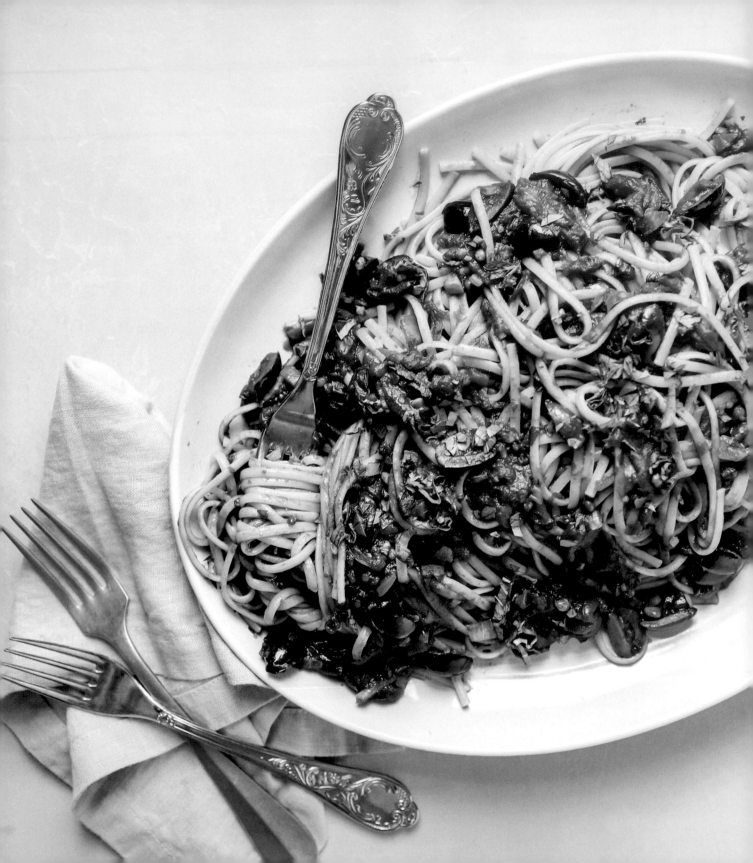

LINGUINE PUTTANESCA

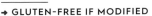

SERVES 4

→ GLUTEN-FREE IF MODIFIED

→ DAIRY-FREE

→ WHOLE30 IF MODIFIED

Total time: 30 MINUTES

Some nights I just want a meatless meal, and when that happens, pasta is pretty much the first thing I turn to—and this particular dish is usually at the top of the list. The recipe has two of my favorite things in life: capers and olives, which is why I just can't get enough of it. If you love salty, savory things, put this on your meal plan ASAP. Trust me, you won't miss the meat!

In a large sauté pan, heat the olive oil over medium heat. Add the onion and cook until tender, about 5 minutes. Add the anchovies, garlic, and red pepper flakes and continue cooking, stirring constantly with a wooden spoon, until the anchovies reach a paste-like consistency, 1 to 2 more minutes. Stir in the tomatoes and red wine (or broth; see Note) and bring to a simmer, using the back of the spoon to loosely break up the tomatoes. Add the olives, capers, parsley, and basil and stir to combine. Reduce the heat to a low simmer and cook, uncovered and stirring occasionally, for 10 minutes. Add the cooked pasta to the pan and toss with the puttanesca sauce. Season with salt and pepper to taste, garnish with parsley, and serve.

2 tablespoons extra virgin olive oil

1 cup finely diced yellow onion

4 anchovy fillets

4 garlic cloves, minced

¼ to ½ teaspoon crushed red pepper flakes

1 (28-ounce) can whole peeled tomatoes (I use San Marzano)

½ cup dry red wine

¾ cup Kalamata olives, halved and pitted

2 tablespoons capers, rinsed and drained

2 tablespoons finely chopped fresh flat-leaf parsley leaves, plus more for garnish

1 tablespoon fresh basil leaves, thinly sliced into ribbons

1 pound linguine pasta (use brown rice pasta for gluten-free), cooked according to the package instructions

Kosher salt and freshly ground black pepper

---

from
MY KITCHEN
to YOURS

To keep this dish Whole30-compliant, substitute low-sodium beef broth for the red wine and replace the linguine with zucchini noodles or spaghetti squash (page 284).

SERVES 4
→ GLUTEN-FREE
→ DAIRY-FREE
→ PALEO
→ WHOLE30 IF MODIFIED
→ GRAIN-FREE
Total time: 20 MINUTES

ROSEMARY-LEMON SHRIMP

- 2 tablespoons ghee
- 6 garlic cloves, finely chopped
- 1 large shallot, finely diced (¼ cup)
- ½ teaspoon crushed red pepper flakes
- 1 large lemon, cut in ⅛-inch slices
- 1 sprig fresh rosemary
- 2 pounds headless, shell-on jumbo shrimp
- 1 teaspoon kosher salt
- ½ teaspoon freshly ground black pepper
- ½ cup dry white wine (substitute seafood stock for Whole30, paleo)

Peel-and-eat shrimp may not be the cleanest of dinners, but boy is it easy and delicious! Cooking shrimp with the shell on has its benefits: First, it protects the shrimp from overcooking, and second, it adds a lot more flavor to the meat. But most importantly, sitting around a table with the ones you love peeling and eating shrimp is a party in and of itself! For this version of the classic recipe, I've added fresh lemon and rosemary for extra brightness and depth of flavor. Don't worry, though—it's still a ready-to-eat-in-no-time dinner!

In a large cast-iron skillet over medium-high heat, melt the ghee, swirling the pan to evenly coat the bottom. Add the garlic, shallot, and red pepper flakes and cook, stirring, until the shallot is tender, about 2 minutes. Add the lemon slices and rosemary and cook, stirring, until the lemon slices soften, 2 to 3 minutes. Add the shrimp, salt, and pepper and cook until the shrimp is halfway cooked through and still partially pink, 2 to 3 minutes. Pour in the white wine and cook, occasionally giving the contents of the pan a gentle toss, until the shrimp are cooked through and no longer translucent, 5 to 6 minutes. Remove from the heat and serve immediately.

from
MY KITCHEN
to YOURS

This dish goes very well with a crusty baguette; however, it goes well with just about anything! For a grain-free meal try it over zoodles, alongside roasted asparagus, or even with a big salad!

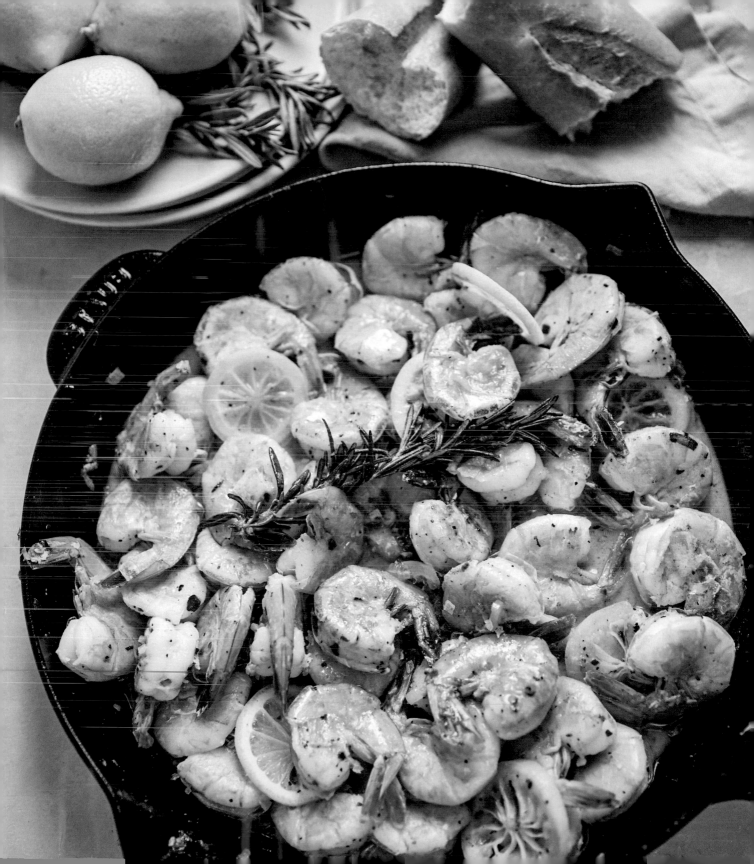

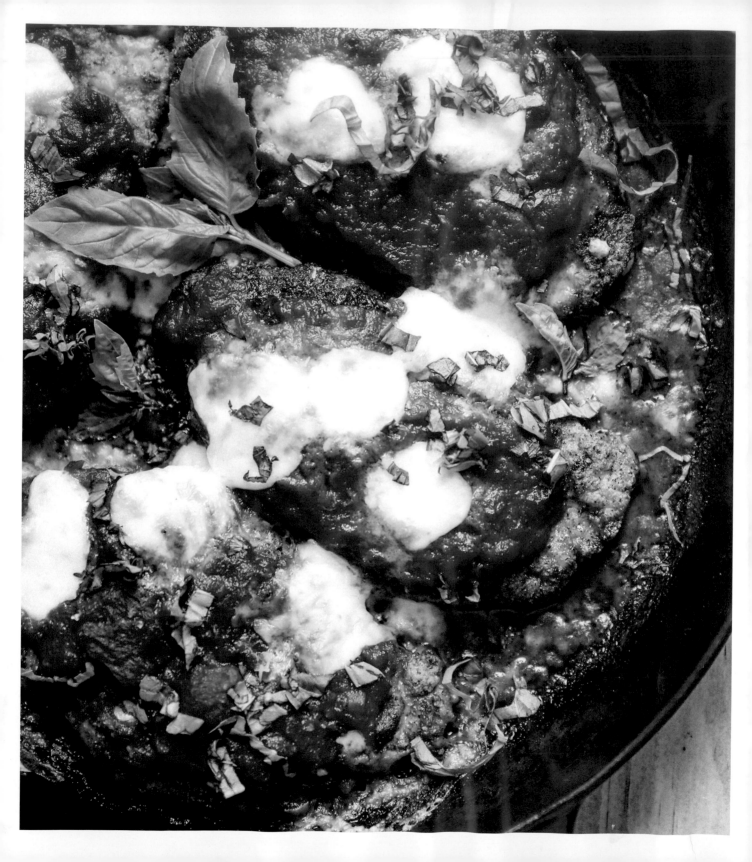

THE BEST GRAIN-FREE CHICKEN NO-PARMESAN

SERVES 4
→ GLUTEN-FREE
→ DAIRY-FREE IF MODIFIED
→ PALEO IF MODIFIED
→ WHOLE30 IF MODIFIED
→ GRAIN-FREE
Total time: 35 MINUTES

"Mommy, this is the best chicken ever! Yummy!" Those are the words that every mom wants to hear at dinnertime, and it is exactly what my little girls told me the first time I made this dish for them. Chicken Parmesan is an Italian classic, traditionally made with chicken that's coated with Parmesan cheese and breadcrumbs. I've given this recipe a grain-free spin (and dairy-free, if you omit the mozzarella topping) so that everyone can enjoy this on any night. Plus, you can serve the chicken with just about anything—gluten-free pasta, zoodles, salad, roasted veggies—and have a wholesome, extremely family-friendly meal.

4 (8-ounce) boneless, skinless chicken breasts

2 large eggs

¾ cup almond flour

½ cup tapioca starch

1 teaspoon dried parsley

1 teaspoon garlic powder

1½ teaspoons kosher salt

½ teaspoon freshly ground black pepper

½ teaspoon paprika

¼ cup extra virgin olive oil

1 cup store-bought marinara sauce (I like Rao's)

1 (8-ounce) ball fresh buffalo mozzarella, drained and torn into 1-inch pieces (omit for dairy-free, paleo, Whole30)

2 tablespoons fresh basil leaves, sliced into thin ribbons

Preheat the oven to 375°F.

Place a sheet of parchment paper over each of the chicken breasts and use the smooth side of a meat mallet (or the back of a skillet) to pound them until they are an even ½ inch thick. Pat dry.

In a medium bowl, whisk the eggs with 1 tablespoon of water until frothy.

In a separate medium bowl, combine the almond flour, tapioca starch, parsley, garlic powder, salt, pepper, and paprika. Stir until well combined.

Dip a chicken breast in the egg and flip to coat both sides, shaking off excess liquid, then immediately dredge in the almond flour mixture to coat evenly all over. Shake off excess and set the

{ continued }

dredged chicken breast on a clean plate. Continue until all the chicken is coated.

In a large oven-safe skillet, heat the olive oil over medium-high heat. Cook the chicken until golden brown and cooked through, 4 to 5 minutes per side.

Remove the pan from the heat and ladle ¼ cup marinara sauce over each piece of chicken and scatter the mozzarella, if using, over the top. Transfer the pan to the oven and cook until the sauce and cheese are bubbly, 12 to 15 minutes. Top with the basil and serve immediately.

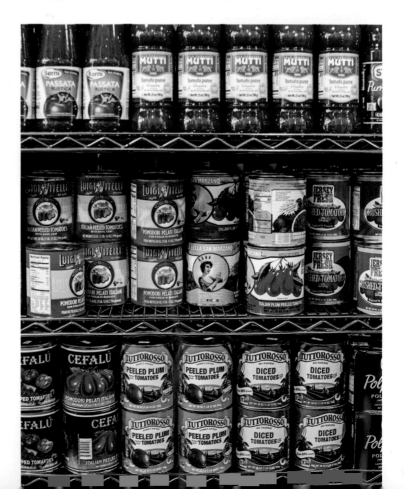

LASAGNA-STUFFED ZUCCHINI BOATS

SERVES 4

→ GLUTEN-FREE

→ GRAIN-FREE

Total time: 45 MINUTES

Growing up, my mom was known around town for her lasagna recipe. It was the cheesiest, most delicious lasagna ever and my friends and I pretty much grew up eating it. We still enjoy it over the holidays when the family gets together, but I wanted to create a healthier version in my own kitchen. While I wouldn't necessarily put the stamp of "healthy" on this recipe, I can assure you that it is much healthier than traditional lasagna without compromising any of its amazing flavors, thanks to using mild-flavored zucchini as a pasta substitute. It's also a great way to add more veggies to your meal. So, no, it's not my mother's lasagna, but it's one I am proud of—and it's perfectly easy to make on a weeknight!

Preheat the oven to 375°F.

In a large skillet, heat the olive oil over medium heat. Add the ground turkey, 1 teaspoon of the salt, ½ teaspoon of the pepper, garlic powder, fennel seeds, oregano, and red pepper flakes. Cook the meat, breaking it up into small pieces using the back of spoon, until cooked through or browned, about 7 minutes.

Add about three-quarters (or about 2 cups) of the marinara sauce to the browned turkey mixture, remove from heat, and cover to keep warm until ready to use.

In a medium bowl, combine the spinach, ricotta, Parmesan, eggs, parsley, and remaining ½ teaspoon salt and ½ teaspoon pepper. Stir until well combined and set aside.

Use a spoon to scoop out the seeds of each halved zucchini to create a "boat."

{ continued }

Ingredients

2 tablespoons extra virgin olive oil

1 pound ground turkey (preferably dark meat)

1½ teaspoons kosher salt

1 teaspoon freshly ground black pepper

1 teaspoon garlic powder

½ teaspoon fennel seeds

½ teaspoon dried oregano

¼ teaspoon crushed red pepper flakes

1 (24-ounce) jar store-bought marinara sauce (I like Rao's)

1½ cups chopped baby spinach

8 ounces ricotta cheese

½ cup grated Parmesan cheese, plus more for serving

2 large eggs

2 tablespoons chopped fresh flat-leaf parsley leaves

4 medium-size zucchini, halved lengthwise

½ cup shredded mozzarella cheese

Pour the remaining ½ cup marinara sauce into the bottom of a 9 × 13-inch baking dish. Lay the hollowed zucchini skin-side down on top of the sauce. Spread about 1½ tablespoons of the ricotta mixture on the bottom of each zucchini boat. Then evenly distribute the turkey mixture between each of the boats. Top the zucchini with dollops of the remaining ricotta mixture and sprinkle all over with the shredded mozzarella.

Transfer the dish to the oven and bake until the zucchini is tender but still has a little bite to it, about 25 minutes. Sprinkle with Parmesan cheese, serve, and enjoy!

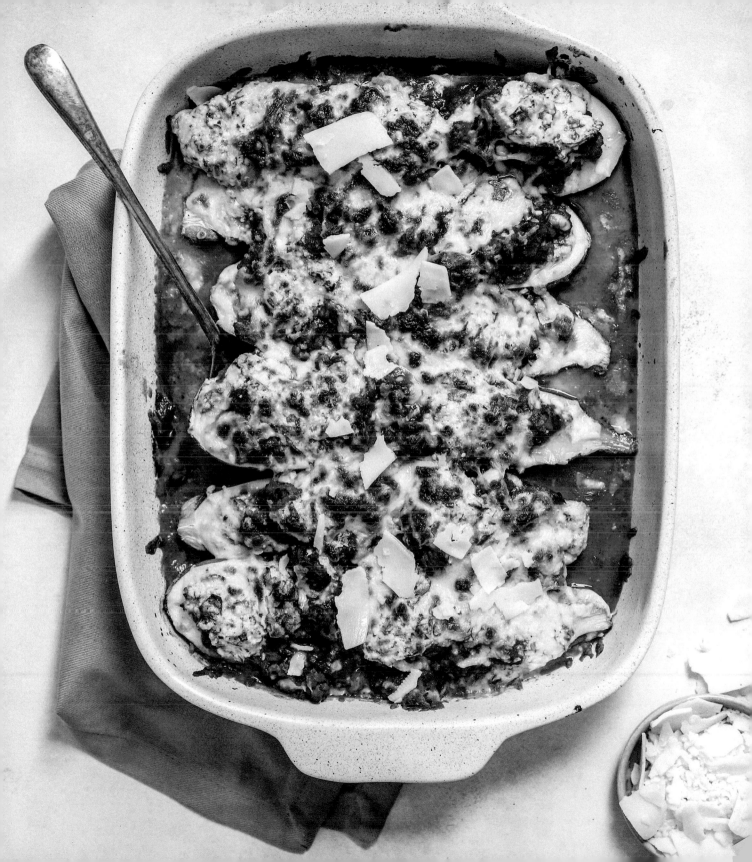

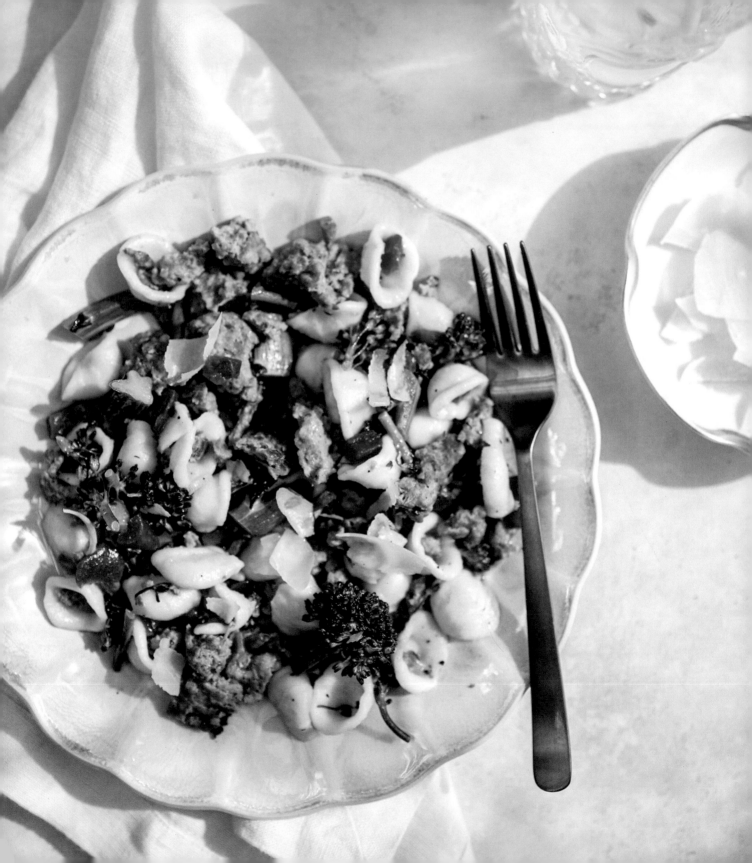

ORECCHIETTE PASTA *with* SAUSAGE, BROCCOLINI, *and* ROASTED RED PEPPERS

SERVES 4

➜ GLUTEN-FREE IF MODIFIED

➜ DAIRY-FREE IF MODIFIED

Total time: 25 MINUTES

It really doesn't get much easier than whipping up a big batch of pasta on a weeknight to feed a family. It gets dinner on the table with little effort, and always fills all the tummies! I love orecchiette pasta, or "little ear" noodles, because the little nooks and crannies catch all the flavors of a sauce. Pairing it with bold Italian sausage, earthy broccolini, and subtly sweet roasted red peppers makes for a fantastic pasta night.

In a large high-sided skillet, heat the olive oil over medium-high heat. Add the sausage and shallot and cook, breaking up the meat with the back of a spoon, until the meat is cooked through and browned, about 7 minutes.

Reduce the heat to medium and add the broccolini and garlic. Cook, stirring occasionally, until the broccolini is tender, 4 to 5 minutes.

Pour the reserved pasta water into the skillet and use a wooden spoon to scrape up all the brown bits from the bottom of the pan. Season with the salt and pepper.

Add the cooked pasta, roasted red peppers, lemon zest, and lemon juice to the pan and toss to combine. Cook to warm the red peppers, about 2 minutes.

Taste and adjust the seasoning with more salt and pepper if necessary, and serve with a sprinkling of Parmesan cheese, if desired.

1 tablespoon extra virgin olive oil

1 pound hot or mild Italian sausage, removed from casing

1 large shallot, finely diced (¼ cup)

2 heads broccolini, ends trimmed and cut into ½-inch chunks

2 garlic cloves, very thinly sliced

1 cup pasta water, reserved from the orecchiette

1 pound orecchiette pasta (use brown rice pasta for gluten-free option), cooked according to the package instructions

½ teaspoon kosher salt

¼ teaspoon freshly ground black pepper

½ cup jarred roasted red bell peppers, drained and diced

Grated zest of 1 lemon (1 tablespoon)

2 tablespoons fresh lemon juice (1 lemon)

Freshly shaved Parmesan cheese, for serving (optional)

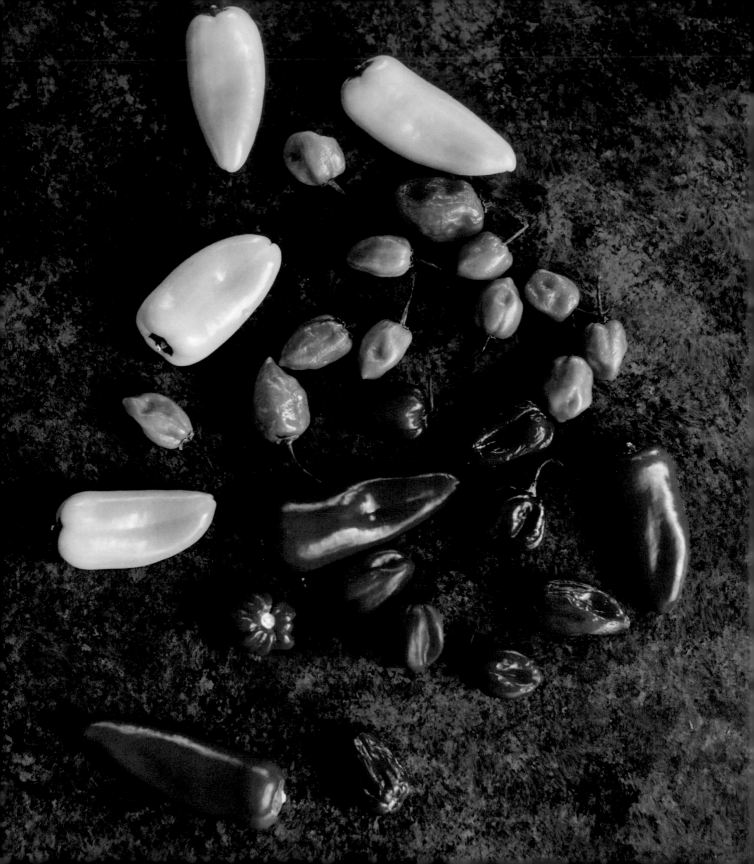

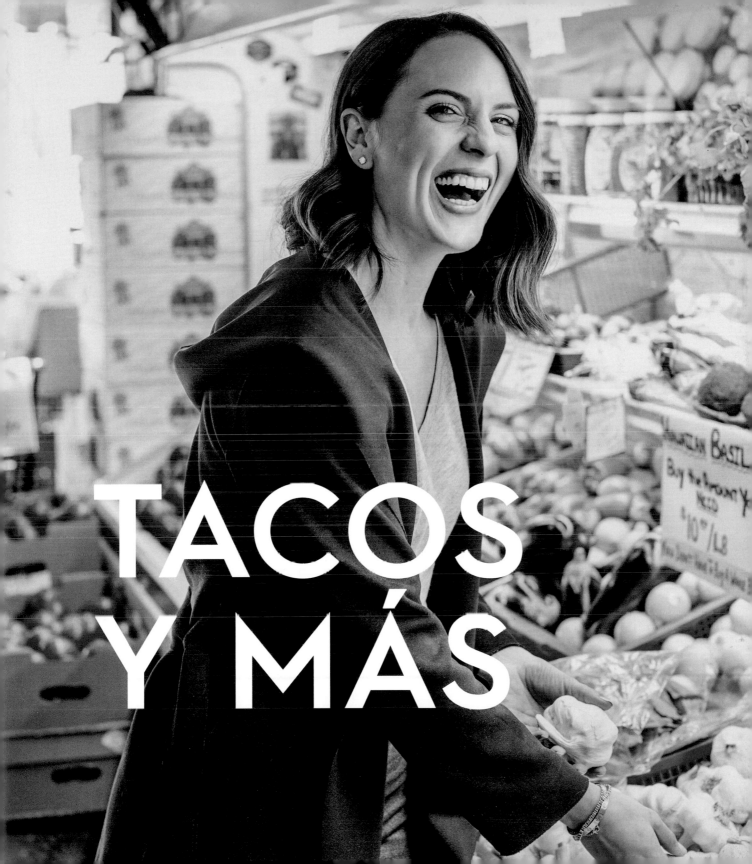

TACOS
Y MÁS

SERVES 4

→ GLUTEN-FREE

→ DAIRY-FREE

→ PALEO

→ WHOLE30

→ GRAIN-FREE

Total time: 30 MINUTES

CHICKEN FAJITA LETTUCE CUPS

FOR THE SEASONING

1 teaspoon chili powder

1 teaspoon kosher salt

½ teaspoon freshly ground black pepper

½ teaspoon paprika

½ teaspoon ground cumin

½ teaspoon dried oregano

¼ teaspoon cayenne pepper (optional)

FOR THE CHICKEN

2 pounds boneless, skinless chicken breasts

2 tablespoons extra virgin olive oil

1 medium red bell pepper, seeded and diced

1 medium green bell pepper, seeded and diced

½ medium white onion, medium dice

Juice of 1 lime

TO ASSEMBLE

8 large butter lettuce or iceberg lettuce leaves

¼ cup chopped fresh cilantro leaves

1 lime, cut into wedges

Because I grew up in Texas, fajitas have always been a big part of my life. Chicken and bell peppers tossed in delicious spices and charred to perfection—I mean, that will just never get old to me! This recipe is my simple weeknight rendition that is packed with flavor and served in crisp lettuce cups to keep things light and fresh. But feel free to use a tortilla if you please! Either way, these fajitas are pretty much the epitome of a quick, easy, healthy, and delicious meal.

MAKE THE SEASONING In a small bowl, combine the chili powder, salt, pepper, paprika, cumin, oregano, and cayenne pepper if desired. Set aside.

MAKE THE CHICKEN Place the chicken breasts on a cutting board and cover with a sheet of parchment paper. Using a meat mallet or the back of a skillet, tenderize the meat by pounding the chicken until it is ¼ inch thick, then cut into 1-inch cubes.

In a large skillet, heat the olive oil over medium-high heat. Add the chicken and arrange in a single layer. Cook the chicken until it is golden brown and almost cooked through, about 3 minutes per side. Add the bell peppers, onion, and the seasoning mixture. Toss to evenly coat. Cook until the bell peppers and onion are tender, about 4 minutes. Add the lime juice and toss. Remove the pan from the heat.

TO ASSEMBLE Fill the lettuce cups with the chicken and vegetables, top with the cilantro, and serve with the lime wedges.

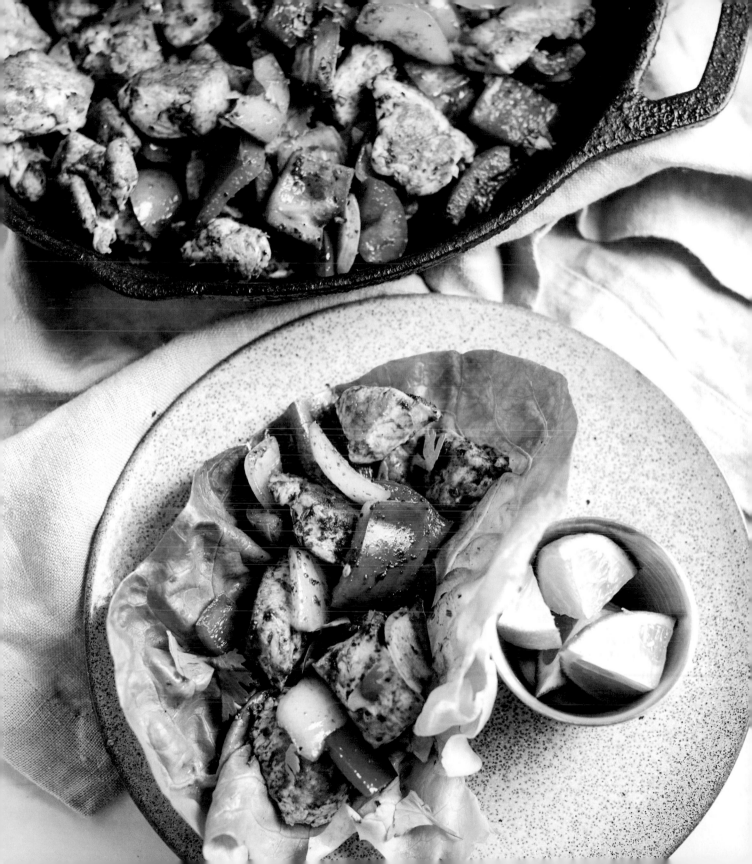

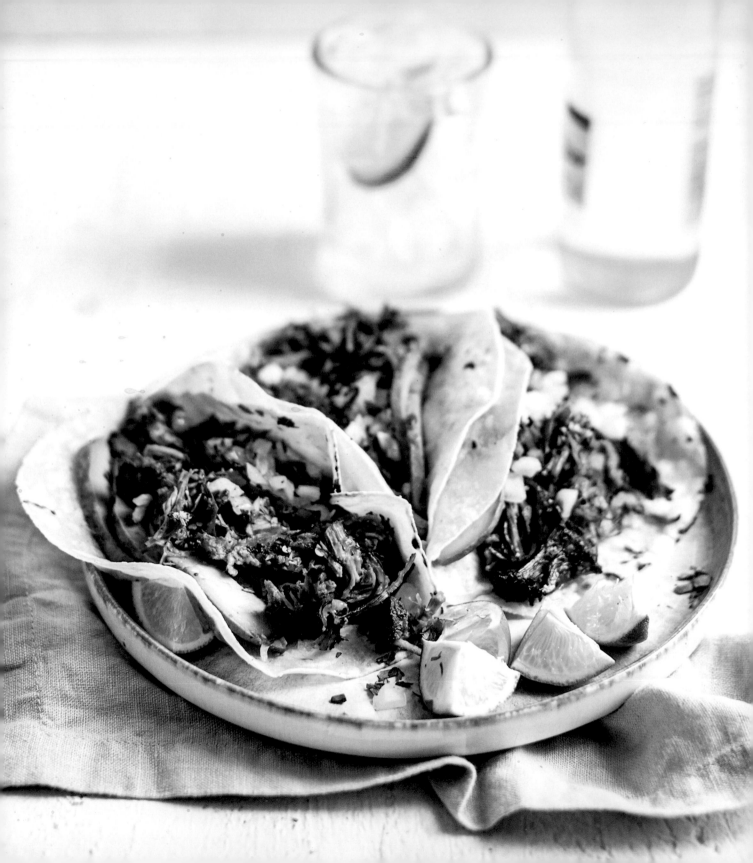

CRISPY SLOW COOKER CARNITAS

SERVES 6

→ GLUTEN-FREE
→ DAIRY-FREE
→ PALEO
→ WHOLE30
→ GRAIN-FREE

Total time: 4 HOURS,
30 MINUTES OR 8 HOURS,
30 MINUTES

Crispy pork carnitas (or Mexican slow-cooked pulled pork) is tender and juicy on the inside and crisp on the edges, making it the perfect protein to put in your tacos. It's also super forgiving: set it, forget it, and your dinner will be ready when you get home from work! All you have to do is pop the pulled pork under the broiler for a few minutes to get it nice and crispy. Happy Taco Tuesday!

MAKE THE RUB In a small bowl, combine the salt, pepper, cumin, oregano, chili powder, and garlic powder. Set aside.

MAKE THE PORK In a separate bowl, whisk together the broth, orange juice, lime juice, apple cider vinegar, and garlic. Set aside.

Cut the pork shoulder into 3 equal chunks. Pat dry, then rub with the spice mixture on all sides until it is evenly and generously coated.

Heat the olive oil in a large skillet, preferably cast-iron, over high heat until it shimmers. Add the pork pieces and sear on all sides, until a deep brown color forms, 2 to 3 minutes per side. Transfer the browned pork to a slow cooker.

Reduce the heat in the skillet to medium and cook the onion, stirring, until slightly softened, about 2 minutes.

Transfer the cooked onion to the slow cooker and nestle them around the pork. Pour in the broth mixture and add the bay leaves. Cover and cook on High for 4 to 6 hours or on Low for 8 to 10 hours, until the pork is fall-apart fork-tender.

{ continued }

FOR THE RUB

- 2 teaspoons kosher salt
- 1 teaspoon freshly ground black pepper
- 1 teaspoon ground cumin
- 1 teaspoon dried oregano
- ¾ teaspoon chili powder
- ½ teaspoon garlic powder

FOR THE PORK

- ¼ cup low-sodium chicken or beef broth
- ¼ cup fresh orange juice (1 orange)
- 2 tablespoons fresh lime juice (1 lime)
- 2 tablespoons apple cider vinegar
- 4 garlic cloves, thinly sliced
- 4 pounds boneless pork shoulder or butt
- 2 tablespoons extra virgin olive oil
- ½ medium yellow onion, sliced (1 cup)
- 2 bay leaves

TO SERVE

- ½ cup finely diced white onion
- ½ cup finely chopped fresh cilantro leaves
- Your favorite hot sauce
- 1 lime, cut into wedges
- 1 avocado, thinly sliced

When ready to eat, turn the broiler on (set to high if you have the option). If you don't have a broiler, heat the oven to 500°F or as hot as you can get it.

Use tongs to transfer the pork to a large rimmed baking sheet. Discard the bay leaves. Do not dispose of the liquid remaining in the slow cooker; reserve it for later. Using two forks, shred the pork and spread it in a single even layer over the baking sheet. Place the pork under the broiler or in the oven and cook until the pork begins to crisp up on the edges, 3 to 5 minutes, depending on how hot your broiler gets. Remove from the oven and pour ¾ cup of the reserved cooking liquid all over the pork. Use tongs to toss everything together and again spread the pork into a single layer. Return to the oven and cook until the edges are crisp, 3 to 5 more minutes. Watch carefully as it crisps to make sure it doesn't burn.

Pour an additional ½ cup of the reserved cooking liquid over the pork and give it one last toss to coat evenly.

Serve with the diced onion, cilantro, avocado, lime wedges, and hot sauce.

from
MY KITCHEN
to YOURS

These carnitas are great served in tortillas or lettuce cups, on top of salad or nachos, or even stuffed inside a baked sweet potato!

CHIPOTLE CHICKEN TOSTADAS *with* PINEAPPLE SALSA

SERVES 6
➔ GLUTEN-FREE
➔ DAIRY-FREE
➔ PALEO
➔ GRAIN-FREE
Total time: 35 MINUTES

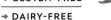

Tostadas are one of my favorite ways to use tortillas. I simply toast mine until they are nice and crisp and layer them high with tons of flavors. I love the layers in this dish—you've got the crunch from the tostada, the spice from the chipotle chicken, the cool avocado, and the bright pineapple salsa. It's one of those weeknight meals that is super easy, but one that will certainly not disappoint!

Preheat the oven to 350°F and line a baking sheet with parchment paper.

MAKE THE PINEAPPLE SALSA In a medium bowl, toss together the pineapple, onion, jalapeño, lime juice, garlic, cilantro, avocado oil, and salt. Refrigerate until ready to serve, up to 5 days.

MAKE THE CHICKEN In a large skillet, heat the avocado oil over medium-high heat. Add the ground chicken, chipotle chili powder, salt, and pepper. Cook the chicken, breaking up the meat with the back of spoon, until it is brown, about 7 minutes. Drain off any excess fat from the pan, if necessary.

Reduce the heat to medium and add the chicken broth and tomato paste and stir to combine. Continue to cook for about 2 more minutes.

Remove from heat and cover to keep warm until ready to serve.

{ continued }

FOR THE PINEAPPLE SALSA

- 2 cups small diced fresh pineapple
- ¼ cup finely diced red onion
- 1 tablespoon finely diced jalapeño
- 2 tablespoons fresh lime juice (1 lime)
- 1 garlic clove, minced
- 1 tablespoon finely chopped fresh cilantro leaves
- 1 teaspoon avocado oil
- ½ teaspoon kosher salt

FOR THE CHIPOTLE CHICKEN

- 2 tablespoons avocado oil
- 2 pounds ground chicken thighs (see Note)
- 2 teaspoons chipotle chili powder
- 1 teaspoon kosher salt
- ½ teaspoon freshly ground black pepper
- ¼ cup low-sodium chicken broth
- 1 tablespoon tomato paste

TO ASSEMBLE
(on following page)

TO ASSEMBLE

    6 (8-inch) grain-free tortillas
       (I use Siete brand)

    2 avocados, mashed

    ½ cup shredded purple cabbage

    ¼ cup chopped fresh cilantro
       leaves

TO ASSEMBLE Place the tortillas in a single layer on the prepared baking sheet. Lightly spray the tops of the tortillas with nonstick cooking spray. Bake for 8 to 10 minutes, or until golden brown and crisp.

Carefully spread the mashed avocado on top of each crisp tortilla. Sprinkle with the shredded cabbage and a big scoop of chipotle chicken. Top with the pineapple salsa and a sprinkle of cilantro.

from
MY KITCHEN
to YOURS

You can also use ground chicken breast, turkey, or beef for this dish.

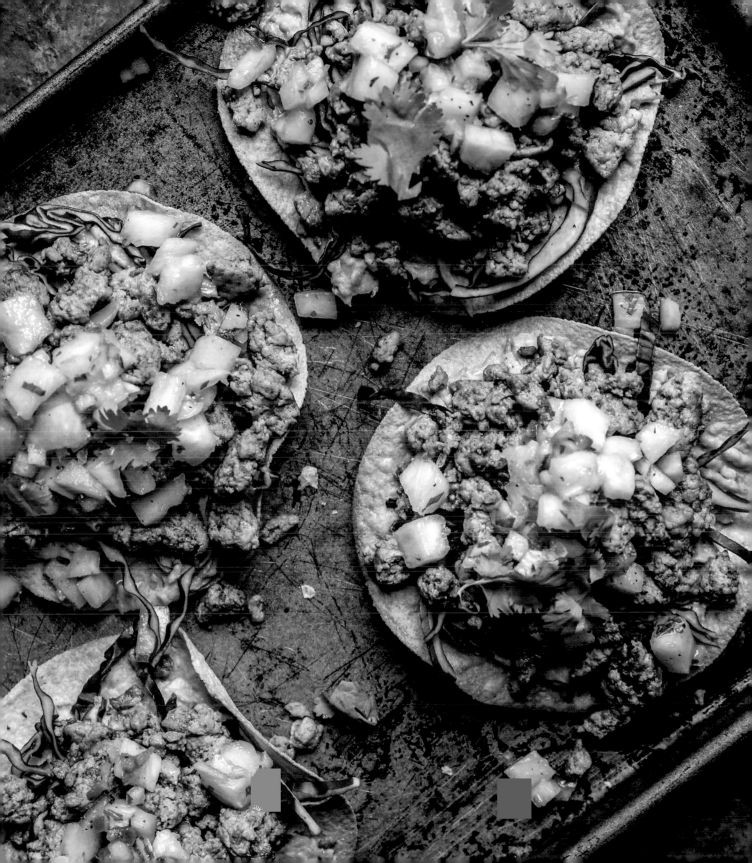

SERVES 4

→ GLUTEN-FREE

→ DAIRY-FREE

→ PALEO

→ WHOLE30

→ GRAIN-FREE

Total time: 35 MINUTES

STEAK STREET TACOS

FOR THE STEAK

1½ pounds skirt or flap steak

¼ cup extra virgin olive oil

¼ cup finely diced white onion

1 teaspoon ground cumin

1 teaspoon chili powder

½ teaspoon garlic powder

1 teaspoon kosher salt

½ teaspoon freshly cracked black pepper

TO ASSEMBLE

1 head of butter lettuce leaves or 8 grain-free tortillas (I use Siete brand)

½ white onion, finely diced

½ cup finely chopped fresh cilantro leaves

2 limes, cut into wedges

Your favorite hot sauce or salsa (optional)

Sometimes the best things in life are the simplest things. This recipe? Case in point! When it comes to street tacos, they are incredibly easy to make and have only a few ingredients. This beef version is one of my family's favorites so it gets requested often, which, as a busy momma, makes me happy because they are super quick to whip up any night of the week. The filling is also just as delicious wrapped up in lettuce leaves if you're looking for a tortilla alternative. Simple, delicious, and classic! You just can't go wrong.

FOR THE STEAK Place the steak on a cutting board and cover it with a sheet of parchment paper. Use a meat mallet to pound the steak 20 to 30 times to tenderize. Discard the paper, then slice the steak into small ¼-inch cubes.

In a large skillet, heat the olive oil over medium-high heat. Add the diced steak and onion. Spread them into a single even layer and let brown, about 4 minutes. Add the cumin, chili powder, garlic powder, salt, and pepper and toss to evenly coat. Continue cooking, stirring occasionally, until the steak is cooked through and slightly crisp around the edges, 4 to 5 more minutes.

TO ASSEMBLE Spoon the beef over the butter lettuce leaves or warm tortillas and serve with the onion, cilantro, lime wedges, and hot sauce. Enjoy!

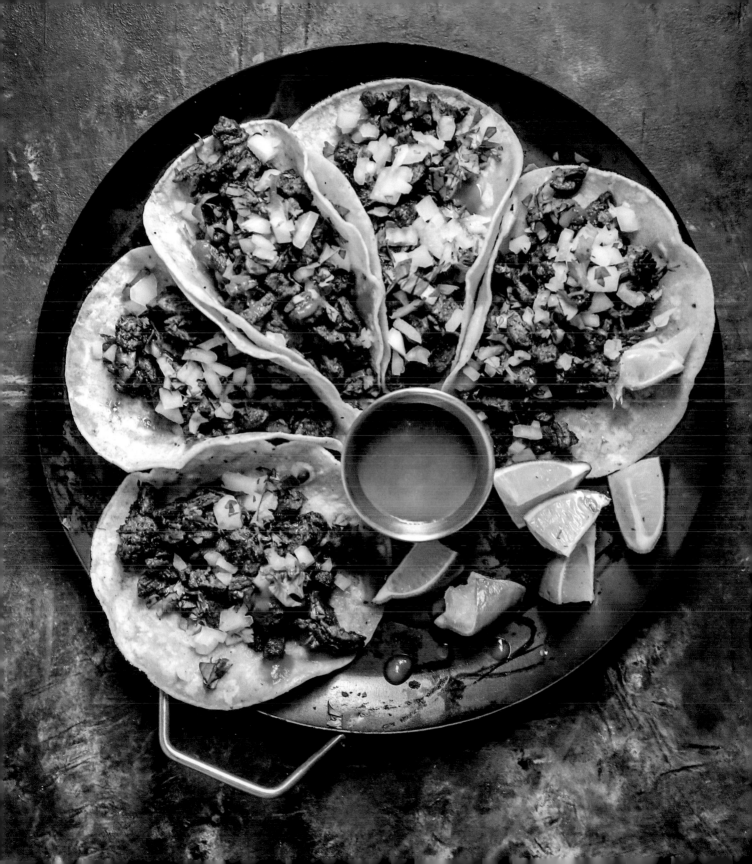

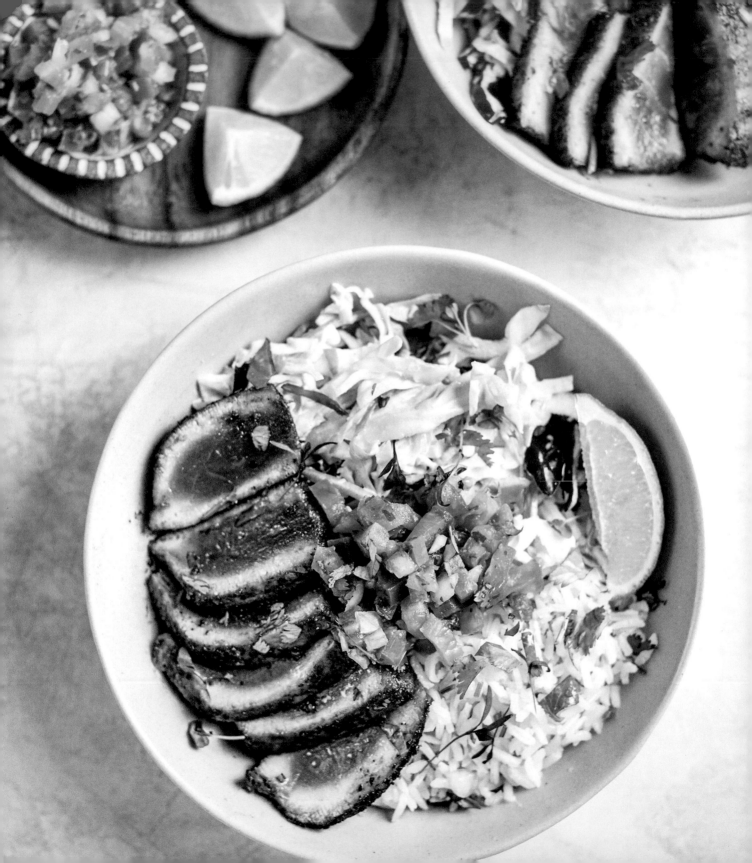

BLACKENED TUNA BOWLS *with* CHILI-LIME SLAW *and* CILANTRO-LIME RICE

SERVES 4
→ GLUTEN-FREE
→ DAIRY-FREE
Total time: 40 MINUTES

I love making this dish when the weather is nice enough to dine al fresco with my family and friends. It's particularly perfect because it requires almost no cooking time (just a quick sear)—so no need to sweat it out over the stove—and it will make you look like a total superstar. Fresh tuna (a superstar in its own right) is rubbed with blackening spices and cooked just long enough to give it a crust but keep it tender and rare on the inside, then tossed with an easy cilantro-lime rice and quick chili-lime slaw. Superstar.

MAKE THE CHILI-LIME SLAW In the bottom of a large bowl, whisk together the mayo, lime juice, garlic, chili powder, and salt. Place the coleslaw mix over the mayo mixture and toss to evenly coat. Cover and refrigerate until ready to serve.

MAKE THE CILANTRO-LIME RICE In a skillet, heat the olive oil over medium heat. Add the uncooked rice and toast, stirring, until fragrant and lightly golden, 4 to 5 minutes, being careful not to let the rice burn. Add the lime zest and 1¾ cups water, stir, and bring to a boil. Reduce the heat to a low simmer, cover, and let the rice cook for 15 minutes. Remove the pan from the heat and let the rice sit, covered, for 10 more minutes. Transfer the rice to a serving bowl and add the lime juice, cilantro, and salt. Toss to combine and cover to keep warm until serving.

{ continued }

FOR THE CHILI-LIME SLAW

- 3 tablespoons homemade mayo (page 281)
- ¼ cup fresh lime juice (about 2 limes)
- 2 garlic cloves, minced
- ½ teaspoon chili powder
- ½ teaspoon kosher salt
- 4 cups store-bought coleslaw mix

FOR THE CILANTRO-LIME RICE

- 2 tablespoons extra virgin olive oil
- 1 cup uncooked white basmati rice (or other long-grain rice)
  Grated zest of 1 lime (2 teaspoons)
- ¼ cup fresh lime juice (about 2 limes)
- ¼ cup chopped fresh cilantro leaves
- 1 teaspoon kosher salt

FOR THE BLACKENED TUNA
(on following page)

FOR THE BLACKENED TUNA

- 2 teaspoons chili powder
- 1½ teaspoons kosher salt
- 1 teaspoon freshly ground black pepper
- 1 teaspoon paprika
- 1 teaspoon garlic powder
- 1 teaspoon onion powder
- ½ teaspoon cayenne pepper
- ½ teaspoon ground cumin
- ½ teaspoon dried oregano
- 4 (6-ounce) bigeye tuna steaks
- 2 tablespoons avocado oil
- 1 cup store-bought pico de gallo, for serving
- 2 tablespoons freshly chopped cilantro leaves, for serving
- 1 lime, cut into wedges, for serving

MAKE THE BLACKENED TUNA In a large bowl, combine the chili powder, salt, pepper, paprika, garlic powder, onion powder, cayenne, cumin, and oregano. Stir to combine.

Place the tuna steaks on a plate and evenly rub the blackening seasoning all over to coat.

In a large nonstick skillet, heat the avocado oil over high heat until lightly smoking. Sear the tuna steaks for 1 to 2 minutes per side, until a black crust has formed but the inside is still rare. Transfer the tuna to a plate and thinly slice using a good, sharp knife.

To serve, divide the rice and slaw among 4 serving bowls and top with tuna slices. Top with the pico de gallo, cilantro, and lime wedges.

COLLARD GREEN *and* CHICKEN BURRITOS

SERVES 4
→ GLUTEN-FREE
→ DAIRY-FREE
→ PALEO
→ WHOLE30
→ GRAIN-FREE
Total time: 35 MINUTES

I love using collard greens to make wraps in my home. You can really get creative and fill them with whatever you have on hand: I do deli meats for grain-free sandwiches, chicken salads for a unique take on lunch wraps, or these hearty but healthy burritos for a fun weeknight meal. Collard greens are great for wrapping as they are sturdy and hold together great. Here, I've veggie-fied the traditional Mexican crowd-pleasing burrito! It's got all of the goodies that are normally stuffed into a burrito, but uses only clean ingredients. The flavor of the cauliflower rice and chicken combination inside is so fantastic, you can eat it alone!

- 4 large or 8 small collard green leaves (see Note)
- 2 tablespoons avocado oil
- 1 cup diced yellow onion (½ medium)
- 1 cup diced red bell pepper (½ medium)
- 1 pound boneless, skinless chicken thighs, trimmed and cut into ½-inch cubes
- 1 teaspoon kosher salt
- ½ teaspoon dried oregano
- ¼ teaspoon ground cumin
- ¼ teaspoon smoked paprika
- ½ teaspoon freshly ground black pepper
- ¼ cup fresh cilantro leaves, loosely chopped
- 2 tablespoons fresh lime juice (1 lime)
- 2 cups riced cauliflower
- 2 avocados, sliced
- 1 cup store-bought pico de gallo

To prep the collard greens, cut off the thick stem at the base of each leaf. Use a paring knife held parallel to the cutting board to shave down the spine of the collard down the middle of the leaf. The spine should be as flat as the rest of the collard leaf.

Fill a large bowl with ice water and set aside.

Fill a large skillet with water and bring to a boil. Once the water is boiling, dip the collard greens, one at a time, into the water for 30 seconds. Immediately plunge the hot collard into the bowl of ice water for about 10 seconds to stop the cooking. (This makes the collard greens less bitter, more pliable, and locks in the beautiful green color.) Transfer the blanched collards onto paper towels and pat dry. Repeat until all leaves have been blanched. Set aside while you prepare the filling.

Heat a large skillet over medium-high heat with avocado oil. When the oil is shimmering, add the onion and red bell pepper. Cook, stirring, until the onion and pepper begin to soften,

{ continued }

3 to 4 minutes. Add the cubed chicken and season with salt, dried oregano, cumin, paprika, and black pepper. Cook, stirring often, until the chicken is cooked through, about 6 minutes. Add the cilantro, lime juice, and riced cauliflower and cook until the cauliflower rice has just warmed through, about 2 minutes. Remove from the heat.

To assemble the wrap, lay each leaf flat with the shaved stem side up. Place 1 cup of chicken mixture in the center of the leaf, leaving 3 inches on each side and 1 inch on the top and bottom so it is easy to roll. (If your collard greens are smaller in size, use 2 leaves and lay the greens parallel to each other so they overlap by 1 inch.) Top with avocado slices and pico de gallo.

To roll, fold in sides and roll like a burrito. Cut in half and secure with toothpicks.

from
MY KITCHEN
to YOURS

Can't find collard greens at your grocery store? You can substitute Swiss chard greens instead! These also keep great in the fridge for 2 to 3 days.

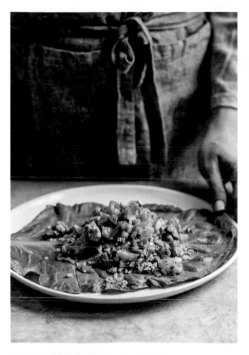

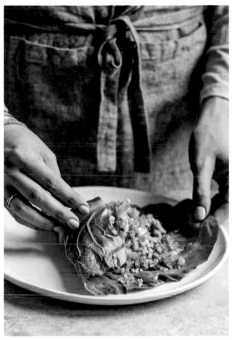

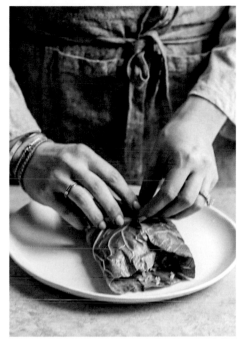

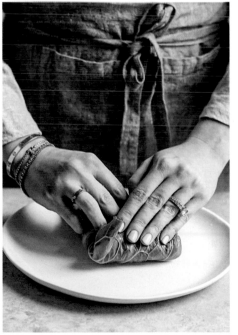

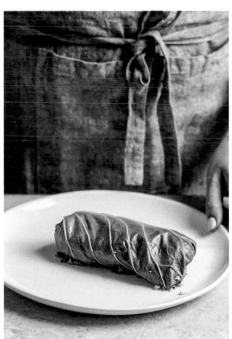

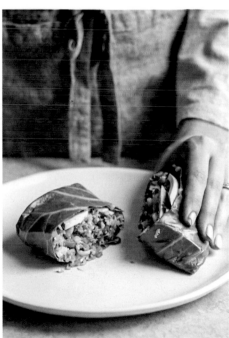

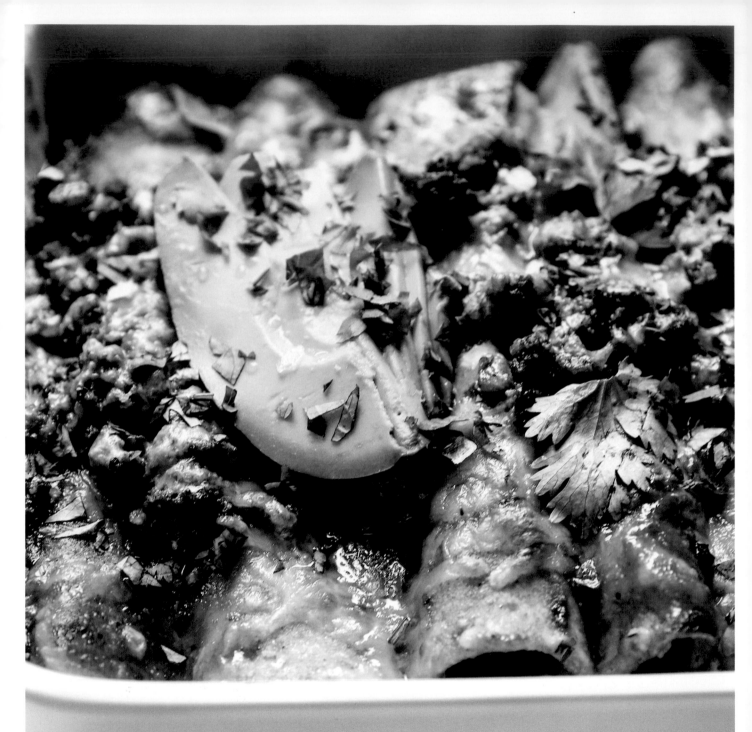

ENCHILADAS
con CARNE

SERVES 4

→ **GLUTEN-FREE**

→ **DAIRY-FREE IF MODIFIED**

→ **PALEO IF MODIFIED**

→ **GRAIN-FREE**

Total time: 35 MINUTES

aka The Best Paleo Beef Enchiladas

Enchiladas always take me back to my childhood and, to be perfectly honest, both of my pregnancies! Seriously, all I wanted to do when I was pregnant with my girls was head to the closest Tex-Mex restaurant and chow down on a big platter of enchiladas. They always tasted great, but I always regretted it afterwards because I knew they weren't the most nutritious option I could have gone for. But hey, when you're pregnant, it's hard to make clear decisions sometimes. The cravings tend to win!

Now that I am not pregnant and don't have the "excuse" to just chow down on a platter of enchiladas on the regular, I had to make my own wholesome—but just as indulgent—version in my own kitchen. These enchiladas are the real deal. I know because, well, I've eaten a lot of enchiladas in my lifetime! And when I make them for friends and family (see Note), I'm told they're even better than the Tex-Mex restaurants in town. Heck yeah!

Preheat the oven to 325°F.

MAKE THE ENCHILADA SAUCE In a small saucepan, melt the ghee over medium heat. Add the arrowroot and whisk just until combined. Add the chili powder, garlic powder, cumin, paprika, onion powder, oregano, and cayenne pepper. Whisk to combine. Continue whisking as the spices toast to prevent them from burning, about 2 minutes.

Whisk in the tomato paste, then slowly pour in 1½ cups of the broth. Cook, whisking constantly, until the sauce thickens, 4 to 5 minutes. Remove the pan from the heat and slowly pour

{ continued }

FOR THE ENCHILADA SAUCE

- 2 tablespoons ghee
- 2 tablespoons arrowroot starch
- 1 tablespoon plus 1 teaspoon chili powder
- 1 teaspoon garlic powder
- ½ teaspoon ground cumin
- ½ teaspoon sweet paprika
- ½ teaspoon onion powder
- ¼ teaspoon dried oregano
- ¼ teaspoon cayenne pepper
- 3 tablespoons tomato paste
- 2 cups low-sodium beef broth

FOR THE ENCHILADAS

- 1 tablespoon avocado oil
- 1½ pounds ground beef, 85 percent lean
- 1 (4-ounce) can chopped mild green chiles
- 1 cup finely diced white onion (½ medium)
- ½ teaspoon freshly ground black pepper
- 8 (8-inch) grain-free tortillas (I use Siete cassava or coconut tortillas)
- ½ cup shredded cheddar or Monterey jack cheese mixture (omit for dairy-free, paleo)
- 1 teaspoon kosher salt

FOR SERVING

- 1 avocado, thinly sliced
- 2 tablespoons freshly chopped cilantro

in the remaining ½ cup of broth and salt. Whisk the sauce until smooth, remove from heat, and set aside.

MAKE THE ENCHILADAS Heat the avocado oil in a large skillet over medium-high heat. Add the ground beef, green chiles, onion, salt, and pepper. Use a wooden spoon or the end of a spatula to break the meat up into small pieces and cook, stirring, until no longer pink, about 7 minutes. Carefully drain the excess fat from the pan and discard. Add ½ cup of the enchilada sauce to the ground beef mixture and toss to coat.

Pour another ½ cup of the enchilada sauce into a wide bowl. Dip each tortilla individually into the sauce to coat both sides, then shake off excess. Fill each tortilla with 2 tablespoons of the meat mixture and carefully roll it up. Place the rolled tortillas in a 9×13-inch casserole dish seam-side down. Repeat until all of the tortillas are filled, rolled, and in the casserole dish.

Pour the remaining meat mixture across the top of the enchiladas, followed by the remaining enchilada sauce. The enchiladas should be completely covered in sauce. Top with the shredded cheese if desired. Bake, uncovered, for 15 minutes, or until the cheese is melted and golden brown and the sauce is bubbly.

To serve, top with sliced avocado and cilantro.

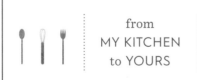

from
MY KITCHEN
to YOURS

This is great make-ahead dish to take to someone in need of a home-cooked meal. I love taking a batch to new parents, someone who lost a loved one, or a dear friend who is a little down. I don't bake it off, but cover it with foil and pop a note on top with directions to bake at 325°F for 15 minutes. They'll be so happy to have a healthy and comforting meal that is made with love.

SPICY RED SNAPPER PLATTER *with* ROASTED ZUCCHINI *and* BLACK BEANS

SERVES 2

→ GLUTEN-FREE

→ DAIRY-FREE

→ GRAIN-FREE

Total time: 45 MINUTES

Here is a dish with all the fixings of a fantastic and festive Mexican-inspired dinner: pan-seared red snapper fillets topped with a spicy sauté of onion and serrano pepper, savory black beans, and simple roasted zucchini. It's a wholesome, filling meal that goes really big on flavor.

MAKE THE ROASTED ZUCCHINI Preheat the oven to 400°F. Line a large baking sheet with parchment paper. Place the zucchini on the prepared baking sheet and drizzle with the olive oil. Season with the garlic powder, oregano, and salt. Use your hands to toss to coat evenly and spread the zucchini in a single even layer over the baking sheet. Roast until the zucchini has started to brown on the edges, about 20 minutes.

MAKE THE BLACK BEANS In a medium saucepan, heat the olive oil over medium-high heat. Add the garlic and cook until lightly browned, about 2 minutes. Pour in the black beans and liquid from the can along with the lime zest, oregano, cumin, and salt. Bring the beans to a simmer and cook, stirring occasionally, until the flavors meld, about 10 minutes.

{ continued }

FOR THE ROASTED ZUCCHINI

- 1 pound zucchini (3 medium), quartered and cut into ½-inch batons
- 2 tablespoons extra virgin olive oil
- ½ teaspoon garlic powder
- ½ teaspoon dried oregano
- ½ teaspoon kosher salt

FOR THE BLACK BEANS

- 1 tablespoon extra virgin olive oil
- 2 garlic cloves, minced
- 1 (15-ounce) can no-salt-added black beans, undrained
- Grated zest of ½ lime (1 teaspoon)
- ½ teaspoon dried oregano
- ¼ teaspoon ground cumin
- ½ teaspoon kosher salt

FOR THE RED SNAPPER
(on following page)

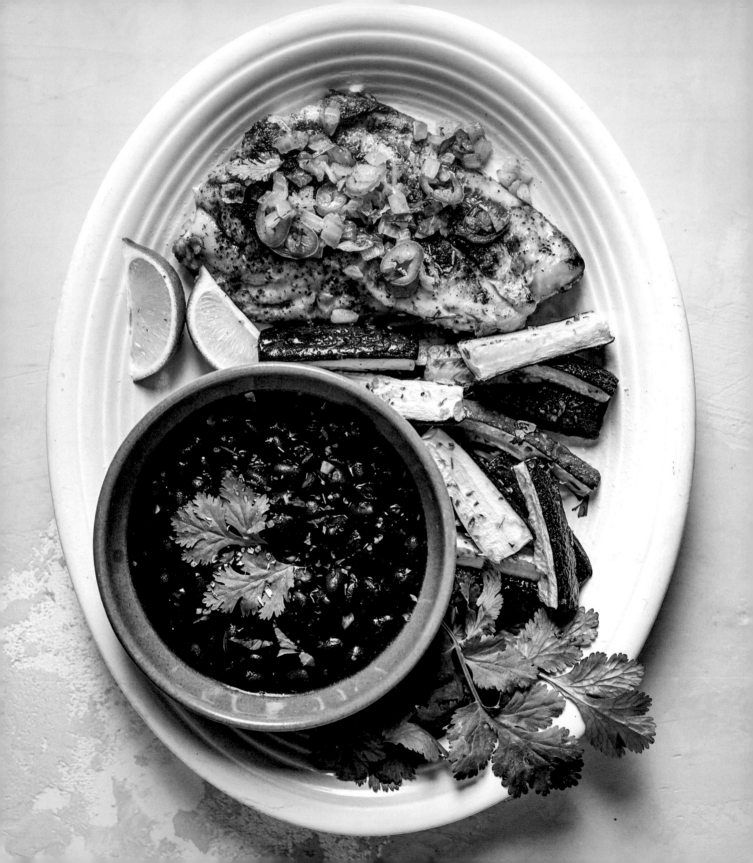

FOR THE RED SNAPPER

- 2 (6- to 8-ounce) red snapper fillets
- 1 teaspoon kosher salt
- ½ teaspoon freshly ground black pepper
- ½ teaspoon paprika
- 3 tablespoons extra virgin olive oil
- ¾ cup very finely diced yellow onion (¼ medium)
- ½ small serrano pepper, seeded and very thinly sliced (1 tablespoon) (see Note)
- 2 garlic cloves, thinly sliced
- 1½ teaspoons fresh lime juice (½ lime)
- 2 tablespoons chopped fresh cilantro leaves, for serving
- 1 lime, cut into wedges, for serving

MAKE THE RED SNAPPER Pat the fillets dry and generously season the flesh side with salt, pepper, and paprika.

In a large non-stick skillet over medium-high, heat 2 tablespoons of the olive oil until it shimmers. Swirl the pan so that the oil evenly coats the bottom. Place the fish skin-side down and press down with the back of a spatula so the fillets don't begin to curl. Cook, occasionally pressing with the spatula, until the fish is nearly opaque and cooked through with just a small raw area on the very top, about 6 minutes. Carefully flip the fish and continue cooking until the top is cooked through and golden brown, about 3 more minutes. Transfer the fish to a plate and set aside.

In the same skillet, reduce the heat to medium-low and add the remaining 1 tablespoon oil. Add the onion, serrano pepper, and garlic. Cook, stirring, until the onion and serrano are tender, 2 to 3 minutes. Add the lime juice and stir to combine.

Serve the snapper topped with the onion and pepper mixture, garnished with cilantro, alongside the roasted zucchini, black beans, and a wedge of lime.

from
MY KITCHEN
to YOURS

The serrano pepper, although small, has a big kick to it. If you aren't into spicy food, I suggest you omit the serrano!

SERVES 4

→ GLUTEN-FREE

→ DAIRY-FREE

Total time: 35 MINUTES

ONE-PAN MEXICAN CHICKEN *and* RICE

2 tablespoons avocado oil

1 cup finely diced onion (½ medium)

1 pound boneless, skinless chicken thighs, trimmed and cut into 1-inch cubes

½ teaspoon kosher salt

½ teaspoon freshly ground black pepper

½ teaspoon dried oregano

1 teaspoon garlic powder

1 teaspoon sweet paprika

¼ teaspoon ground cumin

1 cup uncooked white long-grain rice

1 tablespoon tomato paste

2 cups low-sodium chicken broth

1 (10-ounce) can diced tomatoes and green chiles (such as RO*TEL), undrained

FOR SERVING (OPTIONAL)

1 avocado, sliced

2 radishes, thinly sliced

½ jalapeño, thinly sliced

2 green onions (green parts), thinly sliced

1 lime, cut into wedges

By far, this is my family's most requested recipe in this book. It's easy, full of flavor, and one of those weeknight meals everyone just adores. Plus, who doesn't love a good one-pan meal? Please, if you know that person, let me know, because I need to knock some sense into them. Or I will just make them this dish and change their mind with its fantastic flavor!

In a large skillet with tall sides, heat the oil over medium heat. When hot, add the diced onion and cook, stirring, until tender, about 4 minutes. Increase heat to medium-high and add the cubed chicken, salt, pepper, oregano, garlic powder, paprika, and cumin. Cook, tossing occasionally, until the chicken is cooked through, about 8 minutes.

Add the uncooked rice and cook, stirring, to toast the rice a bit, about 4 minutes. Add the tomato paste, stir until combined, and cook for 1 more minute. Pour in the broth and the can of diced tomatoes and green chiles. Stir to combine and bring to a boil. Once boiling, reduce heat to low, cover, and let cook until the rice is tender, about 25 minutes.

Serve as is, or topped with sliced avocado, radishes, jalapeño, sliced green onions, and a wedge of lime if desired.

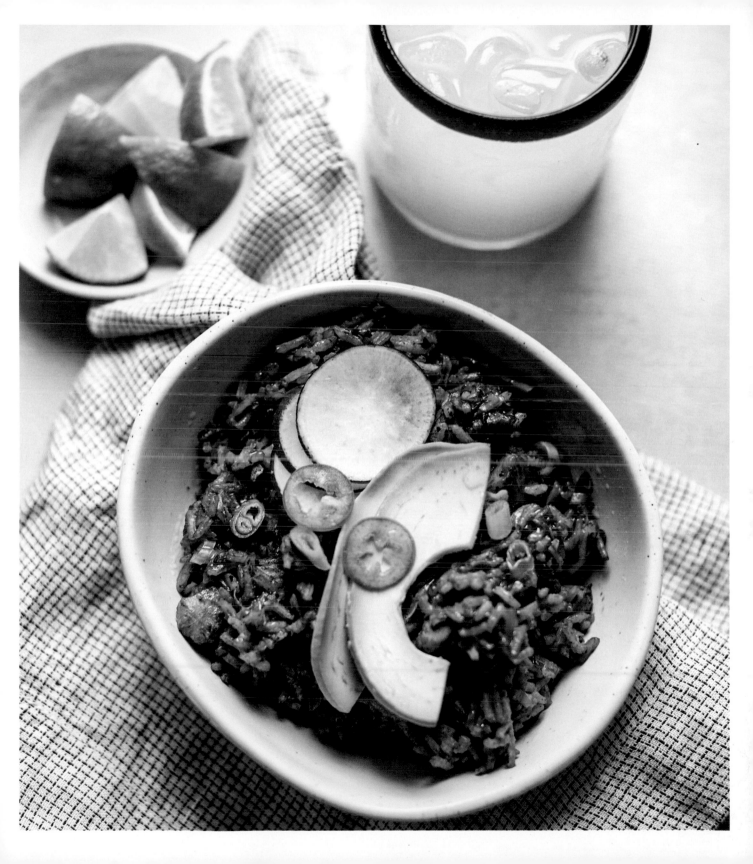

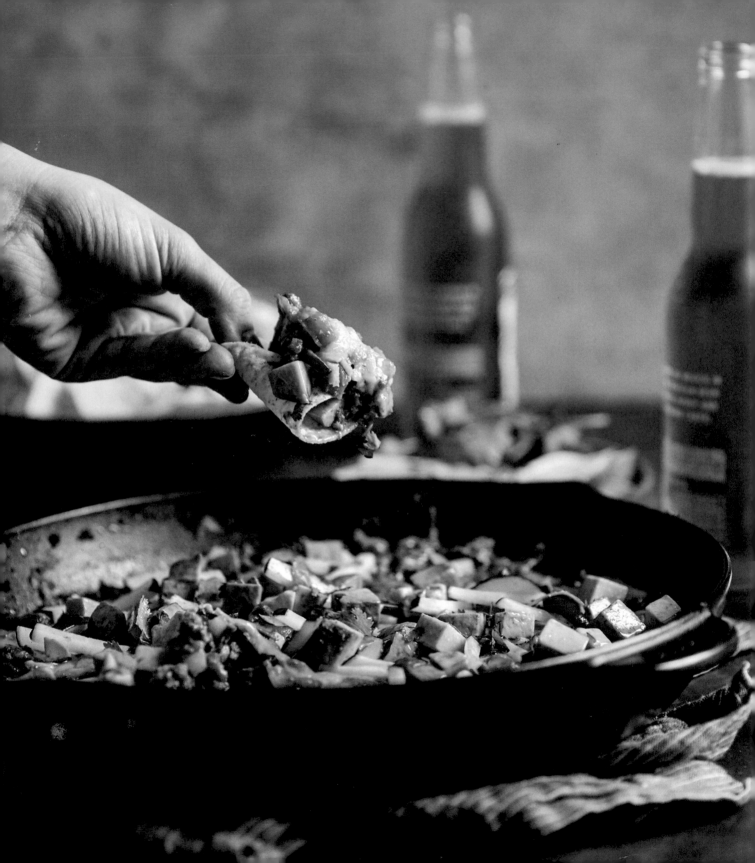

TURKEY TACO
SKILLET BAKE

SERVES 4
→ GLUTEN-FREE
→ DAIRY-FREE IF MODIFIED
→ PALEO IF MODIFIED
→ GRAIN-FREE
Total time: 30 MINUTES

The flavors of Tex-Mex come alive in this super-easy skillet supper featuring ground turkey, lots of chopped veggies, a delicious combination of spices, and a little cheese, all baked until warm and bubbly. I like to just plop the skillet down right on the table so that we can all dig in and have fun with this easy and festive weeknight meal.

Preheat the oven to 375°F.

Heat the olive oil in a large cast-iron skillet over medium heat. Add the zucchini, bell pepper, onion, poblano pepper, and garlic. Season with the salt and pepper and cook, stirring occasionally, until the vegetables are tender, about 5 minutes. Add the ground turkey, paprika, chili powder, oregano, cumin, and cayenne pepper (if using). Cook the turkey, breaking it up with the back of a wooden spoon, until it is cooked through and no longer pink, about 5 minutes.

Reduce the heat to medium and stir in the tomato paste until it is incorporated with the meat mixture. Add ½ cup of the broth and continue cooking while stirring until the broth has reduced, about 2 minutes.

Remove the skillet from the heat and add the remaining ¼ cup broth and stir to combine. Evenly spread the meat mixture across the skillet and sprinkle the top with the cheese, if using. Transfer the pan to the oven and bake until the cheese is hot and bubbly, about 8 minutes.

To serve, top with the diced avocado, cilantro, radishes, and sliced jalapeño, if using, and dig in with chips.

2 tablespoons extra virgin olive oil

1 small zucchini, finely diced (1½ cups)

1 small red bell pepper, seeded and finely diced (1 cup)

¾ cup finely diced yellow onion (¼ medium)

½ cup seeded and finely diced poblano pepper (1 small)

2 garlic cloves, minced

1 teaspoon kosher salt

½ teaspoon freshly ground black pepper

1 pound ground turkey (preferably dark meat)

1 teaspoon paprika

1 teaspoon chili powder

½ teaspoon dried oregano

¼ teaspoon ground cumin

⅛ teaspoon cayenne pepper (optional)

3 tablespoons tomato paste

¾ cup low-sodium chicken broth

1 cup shredded cheddar cheese (omit for dairy-free or paleo)

FOR SERVING

1 avocado, diced

2 tablespoons fresh cilantro leaves

2 radishes, sliced and cut into matchsticks

½ jalapeño, thinly sliced (optional)

1 large bag grain-free tortilla chips (I use Siete brand) or plantain chips

SERVES 4

→ GLUTEN-FREE

→ DAIRY-FREE

→ PALEO

→ GRAIN-FREE

Total time: 50 MINUTES

CHORIZO *con* PAPAS TAQUITOS

1 pound russet potatoes, peeled and cut into ¼-inch cubes

1 tablespoon extra virgin olive oil, plus more as needed

12 ounces Mexican pork chorizo, removed from casing (I use San Manuel brand)

¾ cup finely diced yellow onion (¼ medium)

Avocado oil

12 (8-inch) grain-free tortillas (I use Siete cassava or coconut tortillas)

1 lime, cut into wedges, for serving

Chopped fresh cilantro leaves, for serving

Store-bought salsa or guacamole, for serving

Chorizo con papas, or chorizo and potatoes, is a true Mexican classic and one of my favorites for its bold, satisfying flavors. Although it's great served alone—I love serving it in taquitos because they're portable and fun. Typically taquitos are rolled and deep-fried, but with this foolproof method you can roll them up and bake them for a fun and flavorful weeknight meal.

Preheat the oven to 400°F and line a large baking sheet with parchment paper.

Place the potatoes in a small saucepan and add enough water to cover. Bring to a boil over high heat and cook the potatoes until they are just fork-tender, about 5 minutes. (You do not want them to be too tender, or they will get mushy when combined with the chorizo.) Drain the potatoes and set aside.

In a large skillet over medium-high, heat the olive oil. Add the chorizo and onion. Brown the chorizo, breaking up the meat with the edge of a spoon, until it is cooked through, about 10 minutes. Use a slotted spoon to transfer the chorizo to a paper towel–lined plate. Discard all but 3 tablespoons of the fat in the bottom of the skillet to cook the potatoes.

With the reserved fat over medium heat, add the potatoes in a single even layer in the bottom of the skillet. Cook, gently tossing occasionally with a rubber spatula, until the potatoes are golden, 3 to 4 minutes.

Return the chorizo to the skillet and gently toss until all the ingredients are evenly combined. Remove from the heat and cover to keep warm.

{ continued }

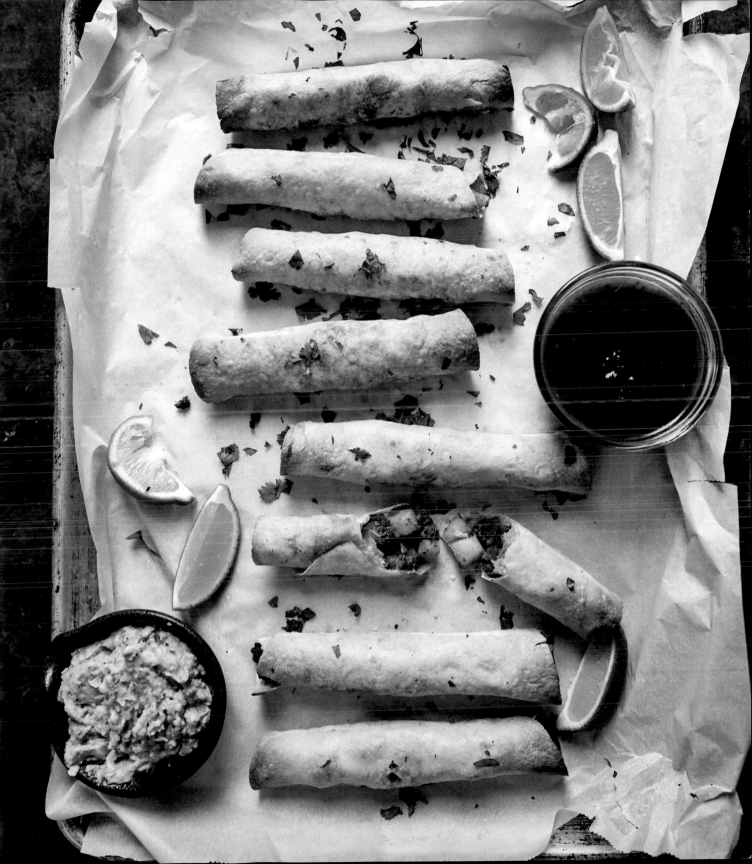

In a small nonstick skillet over medium-high heat, heat about 1 teaspoon avocado oil. Quickly fry 1 tortilla at a time until flexible and easy to roll, about 30 seconds per side. Fill the tortilla with about 2 tablespoons of the chorizo mixture, roll it up carefully, and place it seam side-down on the prepared baking sheet. Repeat with the remaining tortillas, adding more oil to the skillet as needed.

Transfer the taquitos to the oven and bake until crispy and brown around the edges, about 20 minutes. Serve with lime wedges, cilantro, and your favorite salsa or guacamole.

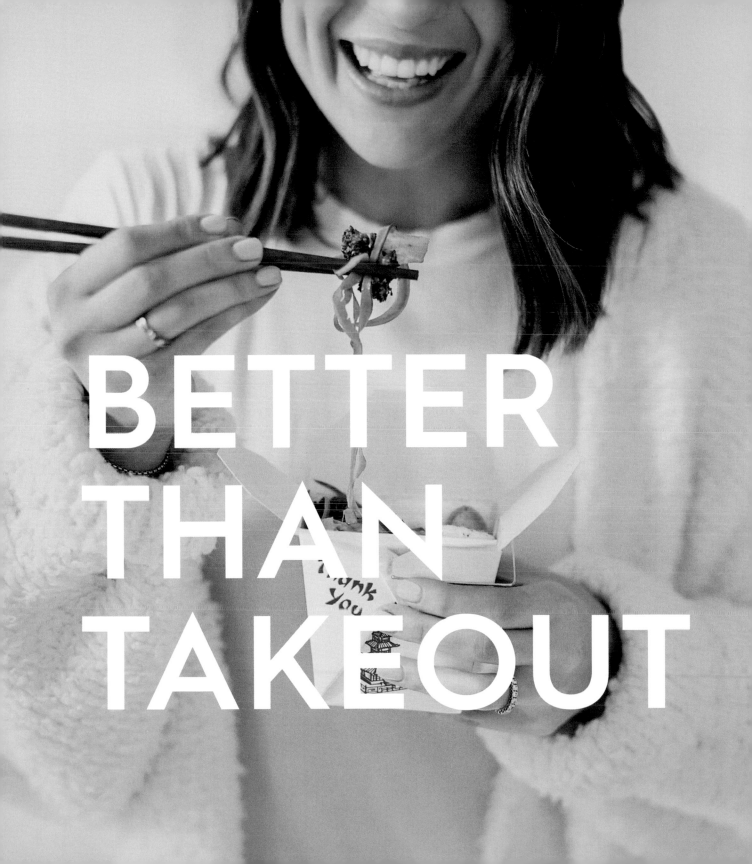

BETTER THAN TAKEOUT

SERVES 4

→ GLUTEN-FREE

→ DAIRY-FREE

→ PALEO

→ WHOLE30

→ GRAIN-FREE

Total time: 30 MINUTES

BLACK PEPPER CHICKEN

FOR THE BLACK PEPPER SAUCE

¼ cup chicken broth

¼ cup coconut aminos

1 tablespoon rice vinegar

1 teaspoon fish sauce (I use Red Boat)

1 teaspoon freshly cracked black pepper (see Note)

¼ teaspoon ground ginger

FOR THE CHICKEN

2 pounds boneless, skinless chicken breasts

¼ cup plus 2 teaspoons avocado oil

1 teaspoon kosher salt

½ teaspoon freshly ground black pepper, plus more for serving

2 tablespoons arrowroot starch

4 celery stalks, ends trimmed and cut diagonally into 1-inch pieces

1 medium white onion, halved and thinly sliced (2 cups)

3 garlic cloves, very thinly sliced

Prepared Cauliflower Rice (page 282), for serving (optional)

You know those days when you look in your fridge to take inventory and think, *What in the world will I do with all this celery?* Well, that happens pretty often on this end. Luckily, when it does, I can turn to this dish, which is one of my favorite ways to get some good use out of that celery. Also, you may recognize this dish from a popular Chinese drive-through chain. This is my much-cleaner rendition that's naturally low-carb, yet completely satisfying. And the decadent and bold black pepper sauce puts it over the top.

MAKE THE BLACK PEPPER SAUCE In a small bowl, whisk together the broth, coconut aminos, vinegar, fish sauce, black pepper, and ground ginger. Set aside until ready to use.

MAKE THE CHICKEN Place the chicken breasts on a cutting board and cover with parchment paper. Use a meat mallet or the bottom of a skillet to pound the chicken until it is an even ¼ inch thick. Discard the parchment, then cut the chicken into 1-inch cubes.

Place the cubed chicken in a medium bowl with 2 teaspoons of the avocado oil, salt, and pepper. Toss to evenly coat, then add the arrowroot and toss again.

In a large, nonstick skillet over medium-high heat, heat the remaining ¼ cup avocado oil. When the oil is very hot but not smoking, add the chicken to the skillet in a single layer (you may need to do this in 2 batches). Cook the chicken until golden brown and cooked through, 3 to 4 minutes per side. Transfer the chicken to a plate and set aside.

{ continued }

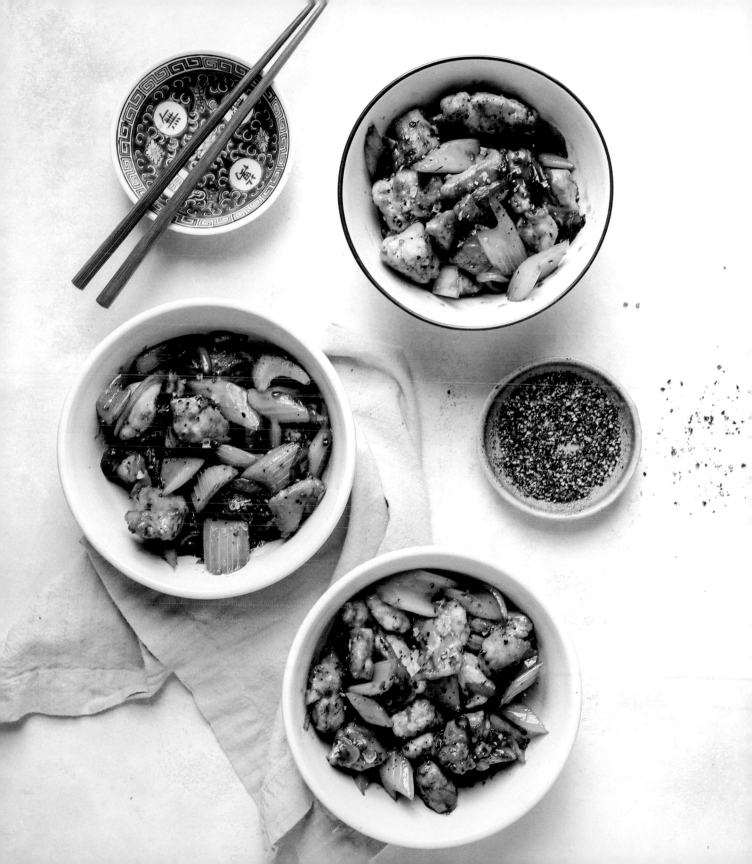

Add the celery and onion to the same skillet and cook over medium-high heat, stirring occasionally, until the vegetables are slightly tender, about 4 minutes. Add the garlic and cook until fragrant, being careful not to burn, 1 minute.

Return the chicken to the skillet with the sauce and bring to a boil. Reduce to a simmer and cook for about 5 minutes, until the sauce is thick and coats the chicken and vegetables.

Remove the pan from the heat and season with salt to taste. Serve as is or with cauliflower rice, and top with a sprinkle of pepper.

from
MY KITCHEN
to YOURS

Regular old ground black pepper just doesn't work in this dish! It's essential that you use freshly cracked black pepper.

THAI BASIL BEEF

SERVES 4
→ GLUTEN-FREE
→ DAIRY-FREE
→ PALEO
→ WHOLE30
→ GRAIN-FREE
Total time: 35 MINUTES

When life gets hectic, a good stir-fry is my absolute go-to because it calls for using just one pan, and typically takes less than 30 minutes to cook. This variation calls for just a few simple ingredients, but it packs serious flavor that will WOW your weeknight.

Place the steak on a cutting board and cover with a sheet of parchment paper. Using a meat mallet or the bottom of a skillet, tenderize the meat by pounding the steak until it is about ½ inch thick. Using a very sharp knife, carefully slice the meat against the grain as thinly as possible. Cut longer strips of the meat in half lengthwise to make them bite-size.

Place the steak in a large bowl and sprinkle with the salt, pepper, arrowroot, and 1 teaspoon of the avocado oil. Toss to evenly coat.

In a large nonstick skillet, heat the remaining 2 tablespoons avocado oil over high heat. Working in batches to avoid overcrowding the pan, add the steak and arrange the slices in a single layer. Sear the meat on both sides until golden brown, 2 to 3 minutes per side. Transfer the cooked steak to a plate and set aside. Repeat until all the meat is cooked and set aside.

1½ pounds flank steak

½ teaspoon kosher salt

½ teaspoon freshly ground black pepper

2 teaspoons arrowroot starch

2 tablespoons plus 1 teaspoon avocado or extra virgin olive oil

½ medium white onion, thinly sliced (1 cup)

1 medium red bell pepper, seeded and thinly sliced

4 garlic cloves, minced

1 to 2 Thai chiles, thinly sliced, or ¼ teaspoon crushed red pepper flakes (see Note)

¼ cup coconut aminos

1 tablespoon fish sauce (I use Red Boat)

1 cup packed fresh Thai or regular basil leaves

Prepared Cauliflower Rice (page 282), for serving (optional)

¼ cup fresh cilantro leaves, for serving

{ continued }

Reduce the heat to medium and add the onion, bell pepper, garlic, and Thai chiles. Cook, stirring, until the onions are very tender, 5 to 7 minutes.

Return the beef to the skillet and add the coconut aminos and fish sauce and stir to combine. Simmer, stirring, until the sauce reduces and thickens, 2 to 3 minutes. Remove the pan from the heat and stir in the basil leaves until they have just wilted, about 1 minute. Serve spooned over cauliflower rice, if desired, topped with cilantro.

from
MY KITCHEN
to YOURS

My kiddos absolutely love this dish, but I serve theirs up before adding the Thai chiles. That way they get a serving that's mild enough for their taste, but the adults can kick things up a notch in the heat department.

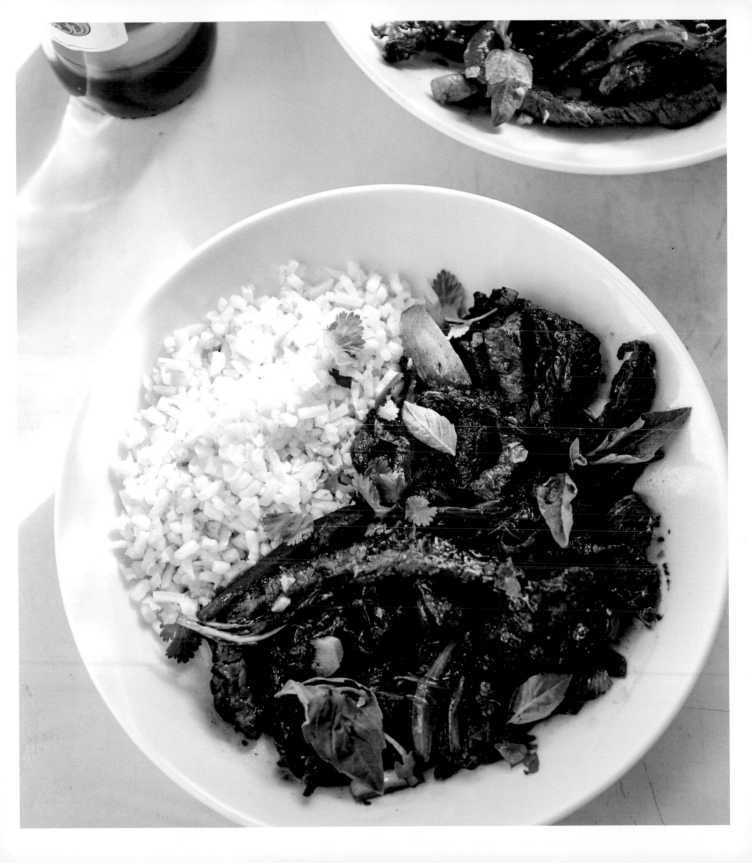

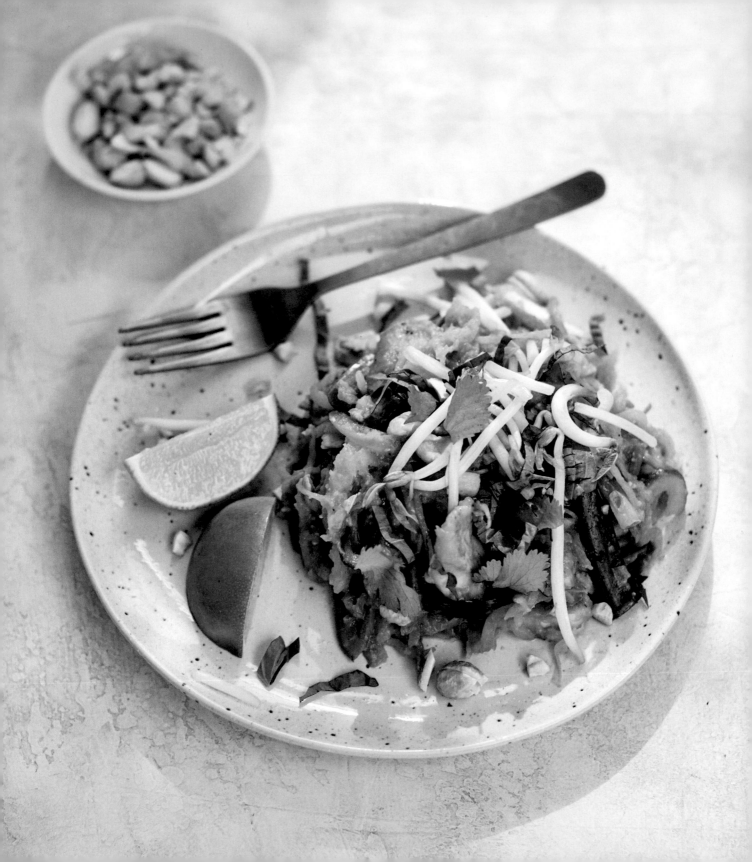

SPAGHETTI SQUASH PAD THAI

SERVES 4
→ GLUTEN-FREE
→ DAIRY-FREE
→ PALEO
→ WHOLE30
→ GRAIN-FREE
Total time: 30 MINUTES
(SEE NOTE)

This hearty dish is a great Whole30-approved take on your favorite takeout pad Thai. Instead of regular noodles, spaghetti squash is the star of the show. Its noodle-like texture not only satisfies the most stubborn of squash skeptics, it also ensures that you get plenty of veggies in your dinner. With all of its delicious Thai flavors, this dish is one of the fan favorites on my blog and couldn't be left out of this cookbook!

MAKE THE PAD THAI SAUCE In a food processor or blender, combine the coconut aminos, coconut milk, almond butter, rice vinegar, ginger, Thai chiles, garlic, fish sauce, and sesame oil. Blend until smooth. Set aside.

MAKE THE STIR-FRY In a medium bowl or on a large plate, season the sliced chicken with the salt and pepper and toss with the arrowroot until well coated.

In a large skillet or wok, heat the oil over medium-high heat until it shimmers. Working in batches, cook the chicken until cooked through and golden brown on all sides, about 3 minutes per side. Transfer the cooked chicken to a paper towel–lined plate and repeat until all of the chicken is cooked.

Reduce the heat to medium and add the red onion to the skillet. Cook, stirring, until the onion is tender, about 3 minutes. Push the onion to one side of the skillet and pour the beaten eggs onto the other side. Let set like a thin omelet, about 2 minutes. Using the edge of a spatula, dice up the eggs and stir them into the onions.

{ continued }

FOR THE PAD THAI SAUCE

- ½ cup coconut aminos
- 3 tablespoons unsweetened full-fat coconut milk
- 2 tablespoons smooth almond butter
- 1 tablespoon rice vinegar
- 1 (1-inch) piece fresh ginger, finely grated
- 2 Thai chiles, thinly sliced
- 2 garlic cloves
- 1 teaspoon fish sauce (I use Red Boat)
- ½ teaspoon toasted sesame oil

FOR THE STIR-FRY

- 1 pound boneless, skinless chicken breasts, cut into ¼-inch slices against the grain
- ½ teaspoon kosher salt
- ¼ teaspoon freshly ground black pepper
- 2 tablespoons arrowroot or tapioca starch
- 2 tablespoons avocado oil
- 1 cup thinly sliced red onion (½ medium)
- 2 large eggs, beaten
- 4 cups prepared spaghetti squash (page 284)
- 1 cup matchstick carrots
- 4 green onions (white and green parts) cut into 2-inch pieces (1 cup)

TO SERVE

1 cup mung bean sprouts

½ cup roasted cashews, roughly chopped

¼ cup fresh Thai or regular basil leaves, thinly sliced into ribbons

¼ cup fresh cilantro leaves

2 limes, cut into wedges

Return the chicken to the skillet and pour in the pad thai sauce. Cook, stirring, until the sauce begins to thicken, 2 to 3 minutes. Reduce the heat to low. Add the spaghetti squash, carrots, and green onions and toss until the squash is evenly coated in the sauce. Remove the pan from the heat and serve immediately topped with the bean sprouts, cashews, basil, cilantro, and lime wedges.

from
MY KITCHEN
to YOURS

This dish comes together very quickly once the spaghetti squash is cooked, which you can either roast in the oven (45 minutes) or in an Instant Pot (8 minutes). See page 284 for both cooking methods.

KOREAN KIMCHI FRIED CAULI RICE

SERVES 2
→ GLUTEN-FREE
→ DAIRY-FREE
→ PALEO
→ WHOLE30
→ GRAIN-FREE
Total time: 30 MINUTES

This dish is one that came about because . . . well, it's all I had in the fridge. Cauliflower fried rice has always been my go-to dinner when the fridge is all but empty, but this time I had some leftover steak along with a craving for kimchi. Combine these three elements together and what do you get? One heck of a meal, that's what! If you love spicy food as much as I do, along with briny fermented veggies, then you'll want to add this to your menu as soon as possible.

Cut the steak into small cubes, about ¼ inch thick. You almost want the steak to look like ground beef. (Yes, this takes a little extra time, but it is worth it!)

In a large skillet over medium-high, heat 2 tablespoons of the avocado oil and the sesame oil. Swirl the pan so the oil evenly coats the bottom. When the oil is very hot but not smoking, add the diced steak, onion, salt, pepper, and chile flakes, if using. Cook the beef until golden brown and crisp on all sides, about 8 minutes total.

In a small bowl, crack two of the eggs and whisk until lightly beaten. Push the steak to one half of the skillet, leaving the other half empty. Pour the beaten eggs onto the empty side of the skillet and cook until the eggs have cooked through and set (like an omelet) about 2 minutes. Use the edge of a spatula to chop up the eggs in the pan and toss them with the steak. Add the kimchi and green onions to the skillet and cook for 2 more minutes, stirring.

{ continued }

1 pound skirt or flap steak

2 tablespoons plus 1 teaspoon avocado oil

1 teaspoon toasted sesame oil

½ cup finely diced white or yellow onion (¼ medium)

1 teaspoon kosher salt

½ teaspoon freshly ground black pepper

1 teaspoon Korean chile flakes or ½ teaspoon red pepper flakes (optional)

4 large eggs

1 cup store-bought kimchi, roughly chopped (I like wildbrine brand)

3 green onions (white and green parts), thinly sliced (¾ cup)

4 cups raw, riced cauliflower

2 tablespoons coconut aminos

1 teaspoon fish sauce (I use Red Boat)

Add the cauliflower rice, coconut aminos, and fish sauce to the pan and cook, stirring occasionally, until the cauliflower rice is just tender, about 4 minutes. You don't want to overcook, or the rice will get soggy. Remove the pan from the heat and set aside to keep warm.

In a medium skillet over medium, heat the remaining teaspoon of avocado oil. When shimmering, swirl the pan so that the oil evenly coats the bottom of the skillet. Carefully crack the two eggs into the skillet and cook until the white is set, about 4 minutes.

Divide the fried rice among two bowls and top each with a fried egg.

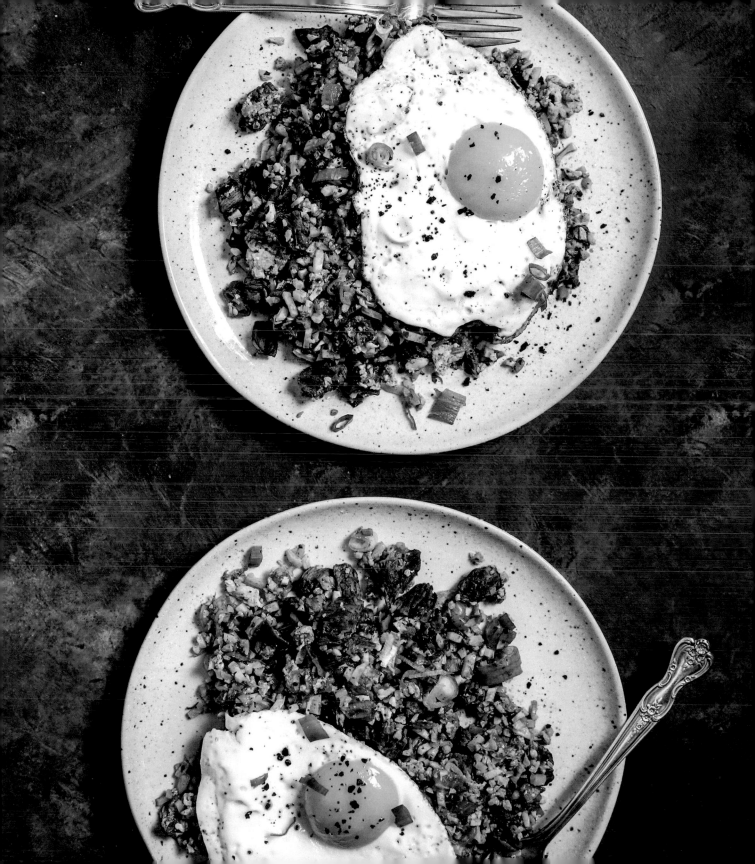

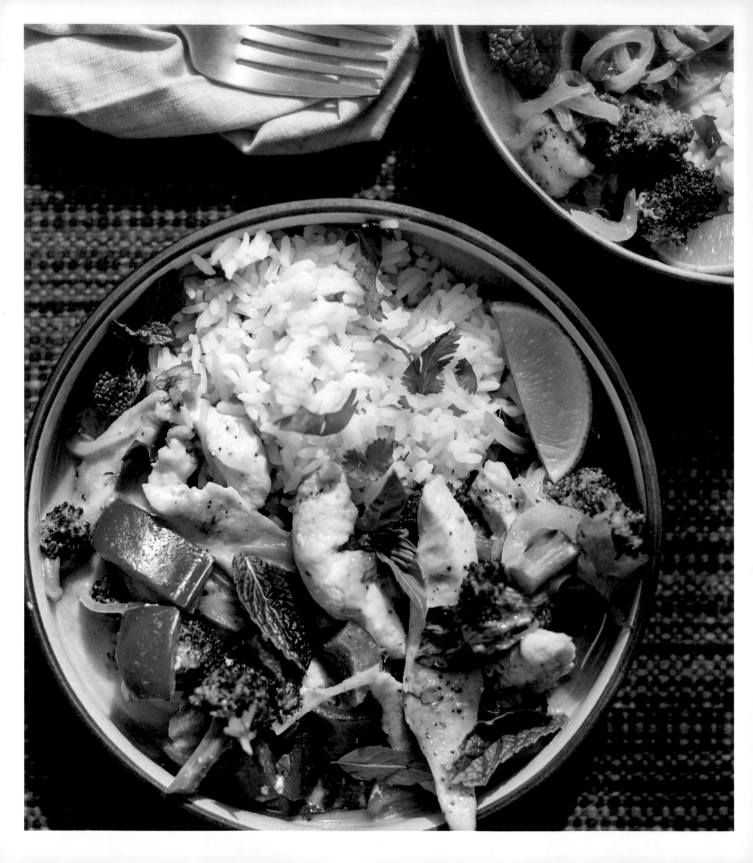

GREEN CURRY CHICKEN

SERVES 4
→ GLUTEN-FREE
→ DAIRY-FREE
→ PALEO
→ WHOLE30
→ GRAIN-FREE
Total time: 35 MINUTES

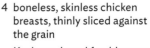

My Aunt Molly lived in Thailand for years, and she introduced me to Thai cooking. The stars aligned, and I have had a serious love affair with the cuisine ever since. When she comes to visit us, she makes a fantastic green curry chicken with sticky rice that I just can't get enough of. Like Aunt Molly's recipe, most green curries are a little soupier, as they are meant to be served with rice. In my version you'll find that the sauce is thicker and packed with veggies, so you won't miss the rice. But hey, if you want to serve it over rice—you do you! It's great either way.

Place the chicken strips in a medium bowl and season with salt and pepper. Add the arrowroot and 1 teaspoon of the oil and toss to coat evenly.

In a large skillet over medium-high heat, heat 2 tablespoons of oil . Arrange the chicken in a single layer in the pan—you may need to work in batches. Cook the chicken until brown on both sides, 2 to 3 minutes per side. Transfer the cooked chicken to a plate and set aside.

Add the remaining 1 tablespoon oil to the same skillet over medium-high heat and add the onion, broccoli, and bell pepper. Cook until the broccoli is tender, about 4 minutes. Add the green curry paste, garlic, and ginger and cook for 2 minutes. Stir in the coconut milk, lime juice, coconut aminos, and fish sauce. Return the chicken to the skillet and bring to a simmer. Add the chicken broth, basil, and coriander. Stir to combine and let the curry simmer for 4 minutes. You may need to reduce the heat to medium-low to keep it at a simmer.

To serve, top with the cilantro and mint and serve with lime wedges and rice, if using.

4 boneless, skinless chicken breasts, thinly sliced against the grain

Kosher salt and freshly ground black pepper

1 tablespoon arrowroot starch

3 tablespoons plus 1 teaspoon avocado or extra virgin olive oil

½ cup thinly sliced white onion (¼ medium)

2 cups broccoli florets

1 medium red bell pepper, seeded and diced

2 tablespoons green curry paste (I use Mae Ploy)

2 garlic cloves, minced

1 (½-inch) piece fresh ginger, finely grated

1 (13-ounce) can unsweetened full-fat coconut milk

2 tablespoons fresh lime juice

1 tablespoon coconut aminos

1 tablespoon fish sauce (I use Red Boat)

¼ cup low-sodium chicken broth, plus more as needed

¼ cup packed fresh Thai or regular basil leaves

⅛ teaspoon ground coriander

FOR SERVING

¼ cup chopped fresh cilantro leaves

¼ cup fresh mint leaves

1 lime, cut into wedges

Prepared Cauliflower Rice (page 282), or steamed white rice, for serving (optional)

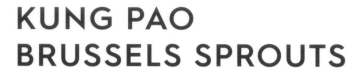

SERVES 2

→ GLUTEN-FREE

→ DAIRY-FREE

→ PALEO

→ WHOLE30

→ GRAIN-FREE

Total time: 35 MINUTES

KUNG PAO BRUSSELS SPROUTS

1 pound Brussels sprouts, halved lengthwise

3 tablespoons extra virgin olive oil

1 teaspoon kosher salt

½ teaspoon freshly ground black pepper

¼ cup coconut aminos

2 teaspoons fish sauce (I use Red Boat)

1 teaspoon rice vinegar

1 (½-inch) piece fresh ginger, finely grated

1 teaspoon arrowroot starch

2 garlic cloves, finely chopped

1 Fresno chile, thinly sliced, or ½ teaspoon crushed red pepper flakes

2 cups cooked rice or 4 cups Prepared Cauliflower Rice (page 282), for serving

¼ cup roughly chopped roasted, salted cashews, for serving

Here are two of my favorite things in life: Brussels sprouts and Chinese food. I love how filling Brussels are, and when they're oven-roasted and crispy? Forget it. I can't get enough! So when I figured out how to make them the star of a dish by tossing them with a spicy Kung Pao–inspired sauce, spooning them over rice (white or cauliflower), and topping them with roasted, salted cashews, you better believe I jumped at the chance—and I didn't miss the meat for one second!

Preheat the oven to 425°F and line a large baking sheet with parchment paper.

Place the Brussels sprouts on the prepared baking sheet. Drizzle with 2 tablespoons of the olive oil and season with the salt and pepper. Toss to coat evenly and spread the Brussels in a single even layer. Roast until tender and browned, 20 to 25 minutes, tossing once halfway through.

In a medium bowl, combine the coconut aminos, fish sauce, rice vinegar, grated ginger, and arrowroot. Whisk until smooth. Set aside.

In a small skillet or saucepan over medium, heat the remaining 1 tablespoon olive oil. Add the garlic and chile and cook, stirring often so as not to burn, until the garlic is fragrant, 1 to 2 minutes. Stir in the coconut amino mixture and let thicken, about 1 minute. Whisk in 2 tablespoons water to thin out the sauce. Remove the pan from the heat. Toss the roasted Brussels sprouts with the sauce and serve over rice, topped with cashews.

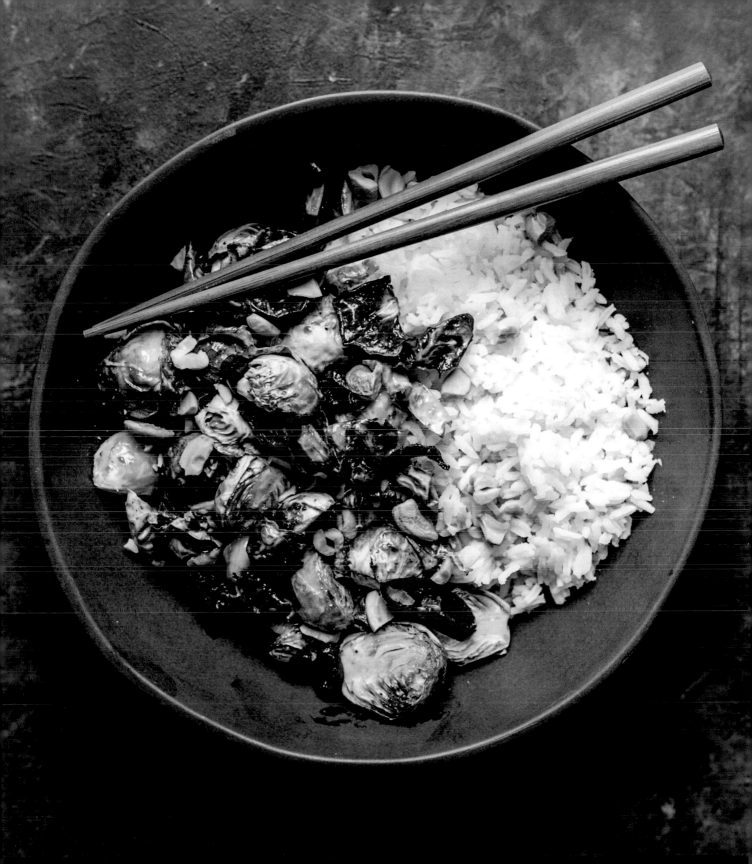

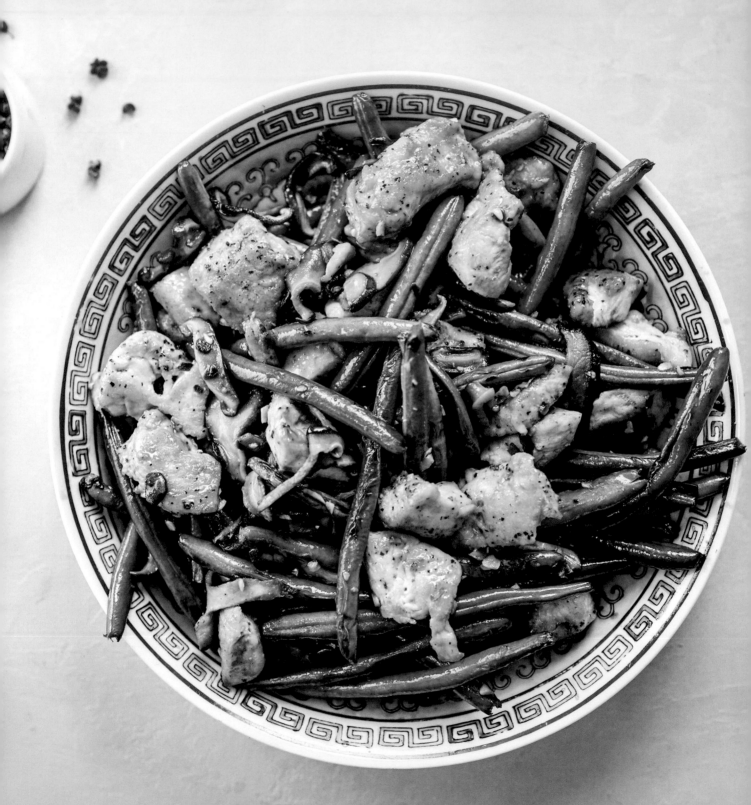

SICHUAN CHICKEN *with* STRING BEANS

SERVES 4

→ GLUTEN-FREE

→ DAIRY-FREE

→ PALEO

→ WHOLE30

→ GRAIN-FREE

Total time: 30 MINUTES

One of my favorite culinary discoveries is Sichuan peppercorns. The first time I tried them in a dish, my eyes grew wide as my mouth started tingling . . . it was an experience like I've never had before and left me wanting more. Yes, Sichuan food is spicy, but don't blame it on these peppercorns—the spice comes from the chile peppers that are also included in Sichuan dishes. Sichuan peppercorns aren't spicy like chile peppers; in fact, they're not peppers at all. They are actually a dried berry from the Chinese prickly ash bush. When you bite into one you may feel . . . well, a little shocked! They make your tongue tingle a bit but, in my opinion, in the most wonderfully addictive way. If it's something you aren't used to and want to give it a try, this recipe will be the perfect introduction. It's simple and with just enough of the tingle to leave you wanting more (and MORE)!

2 pounds boneless, skinless chicken breasts

4 tablespoons avocado oil

1 tablespoon arrowroot starch

1 teaspoon kosher salt

½ teaspoon freshly ground black pepper

¼ cup coconut aminos

4 garlic cloves, minced

1 tablespoon rice vinegar

2 teaspoons fish sauce (I use Red Boat)

1 (1-inch) piece fresh ginger, finely grated

½ teaspoon toasted sesame oil

½ teaspoon crushed red pepper flakes

½ teaspoon freshly ground Sichuan peppercorns (I grind in a coffee grinder)

1 pound green beans

2 cups sliced shiitake mushrooms (about 3½ ounces)

Place the chicken breasts on a cutting board and cover them with a sheet of parchment paper. Using a meat mallet or the back of a skillet, tenderize the meat, pounding each breast until it is about ¼ inch thick. Remove and discard the parchment paper, then cut the chicken into ½-inch pieces.

In a large bowl, combine the chicken with 1 tablespoon of the avocado oil, the arrowroot, salt, and pepper. Toss to evenly coat and set aside.

In a small bowl, whisk together the coconut aminos, garlic, rice vinegar, fish sauce, ginger, toasted sesame oil, red pepper flakes, and ground Sichuan peppercorns. Set aside.

{ continued }

In a large nonstick skillet over medium-high heat, heat 2 tablespoons of the avocado oil . Working in batches so you don't crowd the pan, add the chicken pieces and arrange them in a single layer. Cook until the chicken is golden brown on each side and cooked through, 3 to 4 minutes per side. Transfer the chicken to a plate and repeat until all of the chicken is cooked.

In the same skillet over medium-high, heat the remaining 1 tablespoon avocado oil. Add the green beans and stir-fry until slightly charred, about 3 minutes. Add the sliced mushrooms and cook, stirring, for about 2 more minutes.

Return the cooked chicken to the skillet and add the coconut amino mixture. Cook, stirring occasionally, until the sauce has thickened and reduced, about 3 more minutes. Add salt and pepper to taste, if desired.

from
MY KITCHEN
to YOURS

If your local grocery store doesn't have Sichuan peppercorns, check your local Asian market or you can even find them on Amazon!

MONGOLIAN BEEF STIR-FRY

SERVES 4
→ GLUTEN-FREE
→ DAIRY-FREE
→ PALEO
→ WHOLE30
→ GRAIN-FREE
Total time: 30 MINUTES

This is one of the most popular recipes on my blog, and with good reason! It's hearty, healthy, and one that the whole family can enjoy—picky husbands and kiddos included. You won't believe how much this Whole30 rendition of the classic Chinese takeout dish tastes like the real deal! My first cookbook just wouldn't be complete without this weeknight wonder. Plus, the leftovers are fantastic, too.

Place the flank steak on a cutting board and using a meat mallet or the back of a skillet, tenderize the meat, pounding the steak until it is ½ inch thick. Remove and discard the parchment paper, then slice the steak against the grain into ¼-inch slices. Add the steak to a large bowl and sprinkle with the salt, pepper, and arrowroot. Toss to coat.

In a large nonstick skillet, heat the avocado oil over medium-high heat. Working in batches so you don't crowd the pan, add the steak in a single layer. Sear the steak until it forms a deep brown crust, 3 to 4 minutes per side. Transfer the cooked steak to a plate and set aside. Repeat until all the steak is cooked and all of the meat is set aside.

Add the garlic, ginger, sesame oil, and red pepper flakes to the skillet and cook, stirring, for 1 minute. Pour in the beef broth and bring to a simmer. Let simmer for about 2 minutes and use the back of a spoon to scrape up any brown bits from the pan.

Return the steak to the skillet. Stir in the green onions, coconut aminos, rice vinegar, and fish sauce and bring the sauce to a simmer. Cook, stirring often, until the sauce has thickened, 3 to 5 minutes.

{ continued }

1½ pounds flank steak

1 teaspoon kosher salt

½ teaspoon freshly ground black pepper

1 tablespoon arrowroot starch

¼ cup avocado or extra virgin olive oil

3 garlic cloves, thinly sliced

1 (1-inch) piece fresh ginger, finely grated

1 teaspoon toasted sesame oil

½ teaspoon crushed red pepper flakes (optional)

½ cup low-sodium beef broth

6 green onions (white and green parts), sliced into 1½-inch pieces

½ cup coconut aminos

1 tablespoon rice vinegar

1 teaspoon fish sauce (I use Red Boat)

FOR SERVING

Prepared Cauliflower Rice (page 282)

1 tablespoon toasted sesame seeds

Seared Baby Bok Choy (recipe follows)

To serve, spoon the stir-fry over the cauliflower rice and sprinkle with the sesame seeds. Serve with the Seared Baby Bok Choy on the side.

Total time: 6 minutes

1 tablespoon avocado oil

2 heads baby bok choy, rinsed, dried, and halved lengthwise

1 teaspoon fish sauce (I use Red Boat)

Freshly ground black pepper

SEARED BABY BOK CHOY

In a large skillet over medium-high heat, heat the avocado oil. Sear the bok choy until golden brown, 3 to 4 minutes per side. Add the fish sauce and season with pepper to taste.

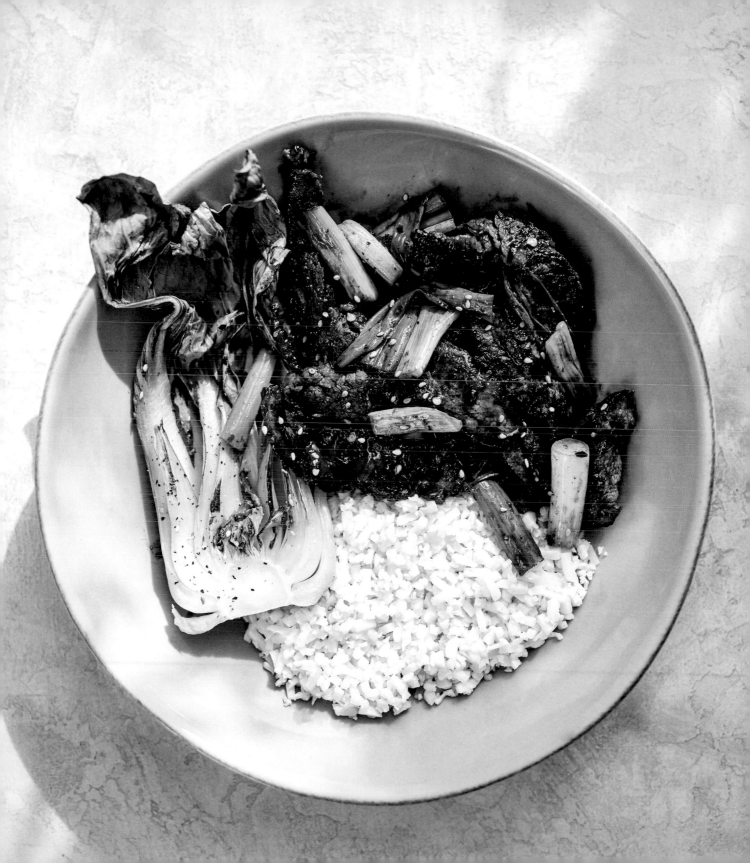

SERVES 4

→ GLUTEN-FREE
→ DAIRY-FREE
→ PALEO
→ WHOLE30
→ GRAIN-FREE

Total time: 30 MINUTES

RED CURRY SHRIMP *and* SWEET POTATO NOODLE STIR-FRY

1 pound jumbo shrimp, peeled, deveined, and tail-off

1 teaspoon kosher salt

½ teaspoon freshly ground black pepper

4 tablespoons avocado oil

3 cups small florets of broccoli (1 small head)

1 cup finely diced red bell pepper (1 medium)

1 pound spiralized sweet potato (1 large)

2 tablespoons red curry paste (I use Mae Ploy)

1 (13-ounce) can unsweetened full-fat coconut milk

1 teaspoon fish sauce (I use Red Boat)

2 tablespoons fresh cilantro leaves

If you do not already own a spiralizer and are trying to make healthier habits in your home, I can't encourage you enough to invest in one. It's a simple and fun way to incorporate more vegetables into your day-to-day cooking. You can spiralize just about everything into noodles, and sweet potatoes are definitely one of my favorite veggies to do that with. In this dish, the sweet potatoes bring a nice touch of sweetness to the heat in the red curry paste. Plus, they make this dish a little heartier to keep you satisfied longer.

Season the shrimp with salt and pepper.

In a large skillet over medium-high heat, heat 2 tablespoons of the oil. When shimmering, add the shrimp to the skillet in a single layer and sear until cooked through and golden brown, 2 to 3 minutes per side. (You may need to do this in batches depending on the size of your skillet.) Transfer the cooked shrimp to a plate and set aside.

Add another 1 tablespoon oil to the skillet along with the broccoli florets and red bell pepper. Cook, stirring, for 2 minutes, then add ¼ cup water. Continue sautéing the veggies until the water has completely evaporated and the veggies are tender, 3 to 4 minutes.

Add the remaining 1 tablespoon oil to the skillet and the spiralized sweet potato and cook, stirring, until just tender, about 4 minutes. Transfer the cooked sweet potato and veggies onto the plate with the shrimp and set aside.

{ continued }

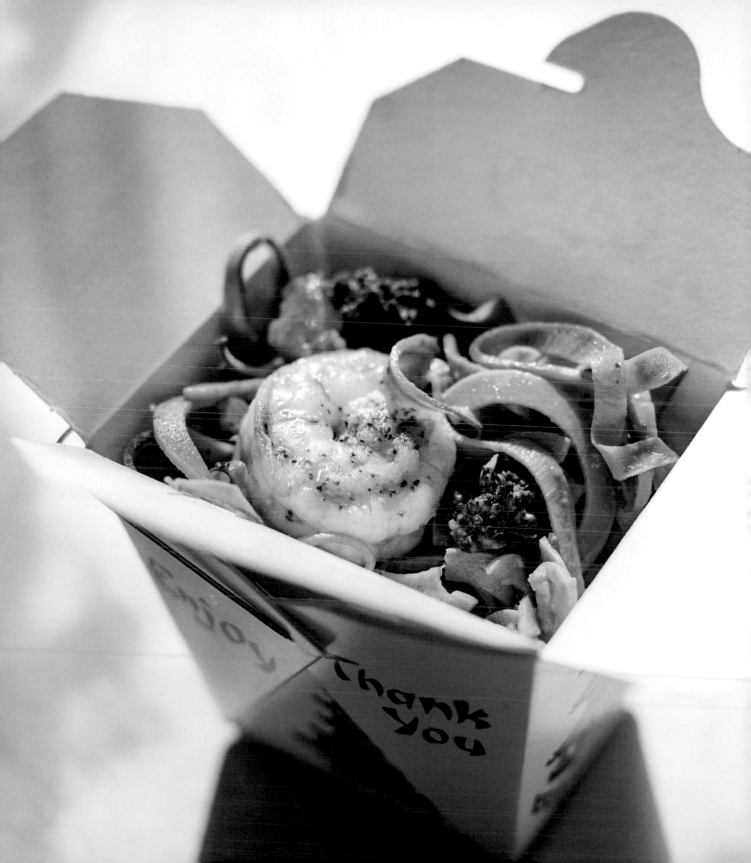

If the skillet is dry, add 1 more teaspoon oil along with the red curry paste. Cook the red curry paste, stirring, until fragrant, about 1 minute. Pour in the coconut milk and whisk to combine with the curry paste. Bring to a simmer. Once simmering, add the fish sauce, then the cooked veggies and shrimp back into the skillet, and toss until evenly coated.

Stir in the cilantro and serve immediately.

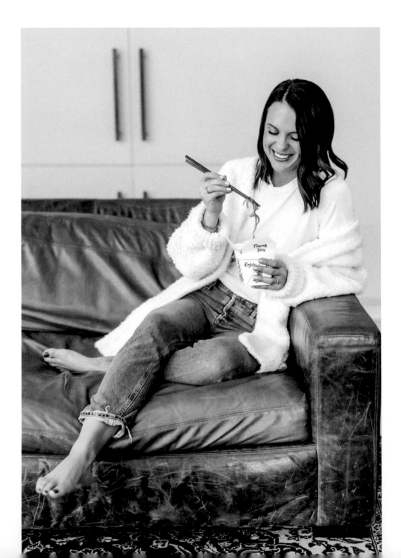

SALMON SATAY LETTUCE CUPS

SERVES 4
→ GLUTEN-FREE
→ DAIRY-FREE
→ PALEO
→ WHOLE30
→ GRAIN-FREE
Total time: 40 MINUTES (PLUS MARINATING)

I absolutely love any sort of satay. If you've never had satay before, it's small pieces of protein grilled on a skewer and served with a spiced sauce that typically contains peanuts. To keep this peanut-free, I've used a creamy almond butter and made a sauce that is absolutely delightful. The sauce is dense and filling, but paired with salmon in light and crispy lettuce leaves, it's a combination that's just irresistible, especially in the summertime!

MARINATE THE SALMON In a large bowl, whisk together the coconut milk, red curry paste, coconut aminos, and fish sauce. Add the cubed salmon and gently toss to evenly coat. Cover the bowl with plastic wrap and refrigerate for at least 4 hours or up to 24 hours.

MAKE THE ALMOND SAUCE In a food processor or blender, combine the coconut milk, almond butter, coconut aminos, lime juice, fish sauce, red curry paste, and garlic. Blend until smooth and set aside.

ASSEMBLE THE SKEWERS Preheat the grill over medium-high heat.

Thread about 5 pieces of the marinated salmon onto two parallel wooden skewers. Continue until all of the salmon has been skewered. Using a pair of tongs, carefully transfer the salmon skewers to the grill and cook until the salmon is fully cooked through, 3 to 4 minutes per side. Remove the skewers from the grill and let them rest for about 5 minutes.

{ continued }

FOR THE SALMON

- ½ cup unsweetened full-fat coconut milk
- 2 tablespoons red curry paste (I use Mae Ploy)
- 2 tablespoons coconut aminos
- 2 teaspoons fish sauce (I use Red Boat)
- 2 pounds salmon (at least 1 inch thick), skin removed and cut into 1-inch cubes
- 16 (6-inch) wooden skewers, soaked in water for 1 hour before using

FOR THE SPICY ALMOND SAUCE

- ¼ cup unsweetened full-fat coconut milk
- 3 tablespoons creamy almond butter (or any creamy nut butter of your choice)
- 1 tablespoon coconut aminos
- 1 tablespoon fresh lime juice (½ lime)
- 2 teaspoons fish sauce (I use Red Boat)
- 1 teaspoon red curry paste
- 1 garlic clove

TO ASSEMBLE
(on following page)

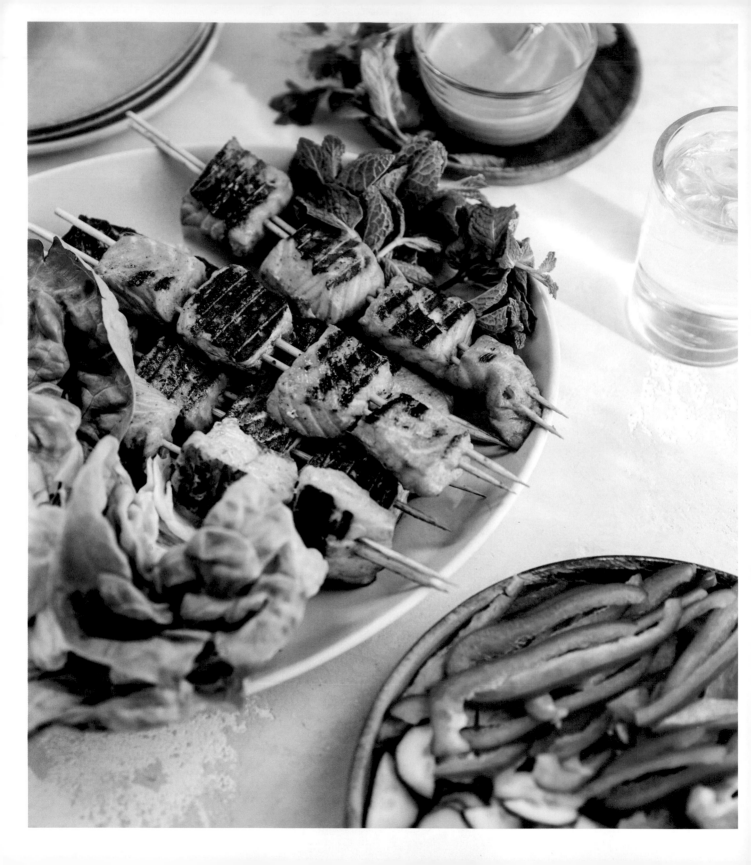

TO ASSEMBLE

8 large butter lettuce leaves

½ cup shredded red cabbage

1 medium red bell pepper, seeded and very thinly sliced

1 English cucumber, halved and thinly sliced into half moons

¼ cup fresh mint leaves, torn into pieces

¼ cup fresh cilantro leaves, torn into pieces

1 lime, cut into wedges

ASSEMBLE THE LETTUCE CUPS Fill each lettuce leaf with the cabbage, bell pepper, cucumber, mint, and cilantro. Gently remove the salmon from the skewers and add to the wraps. Drizzle with the spicy almond sauce and serve with lime wedges.

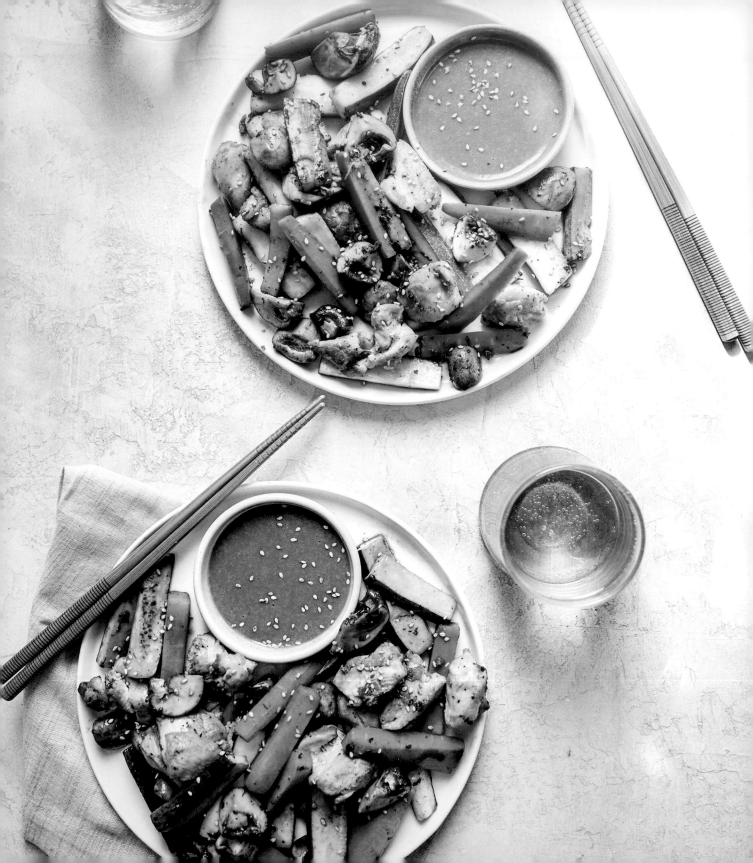

HIBACHI-STYLE CHICKEN *with* MAGIC MUSTARD SAUCE

SERVES 4
→ GLUTEN-FREE
→ DAIRY-FREE
→ PALEO
→ WHOLE30
→ GRAIN-FREE
Total time: 30 MINUTES

Raise your hand if you grew up celebrating all of your teen birthdays at a hibachi-style restaurant! Ah, a hand over here is raised high and I am not mad about it. The little food lover in me used to love watching the chefs fry rice right at the table, and I'd always take mental note of all the ingredients they used so I could go home and re-create the meal. If you are like me and spent many a birthday enjoying tableside fried rice, I know you know about that magical mustard sauce they set in front of you. Served with both red and white meat, this mustard sauce has unique flavors of salty, sour, and tangy all at once that elevate flavor way beyond traditional Chinese mustard. Good grief, the stuff is so good! I just had to remake it in my own kitchen, and when I shared this on my blog, it quickly became one of the top ranked recipes—which means it had to be in this cookbook! So fire up your woks, bring the hibachi experience into your own home, and have some good old-fashioned fun!

MAKE THE MAGIC MUSTARD SAUCE In a small bowl, whisk together the mustard powder and 2 tablespoons of warm water. Add the mixture to a food processor and combine with the coconut aminos, tahini, ginger, garlic, and fish sauce. Blend until smooth. Set aside.

MAKE THE STIR-FRY Place the cubed chicken in a large bowl and toss with the salt and pepper to evenly coat.

{ continued }

**FOR THE MAGIC
MUSTARD SAUCE**

  2 teaspoons mustard powder

  ½ cup coconut aminos

  3 tablespoons tahini

  1 (½-inch) piece fresh ginger, finely grated

  2 garlic cloves

  1 teaspoon fish sauce (I use Red Boat)

FOR THE STIR-FRY

  2 pounds boneless, skinless chicken thighs, trimmed and cut into 1-inch cubes

  ½ teaspoon kosher salt

      Freshly ground black pepper

  2 tablespoons avocado oil

  1 tablespoon ghee

  ½ medium white onion, thinly sliced (1 cup)

  8 baby bella mushrooms, stems removed and quartered

  2 small zucchini, cut in half across the middle, then each half quartered lengthwise

  2 small carrots, cut in half across the middle, then each half quartered lengthwise

  1 tablespoon toasted sesame seeds

In a wok or large skillet, heat the avocado oil over high heat until just smoking. Working in batches so you don't crowd the pan, add the chicken in a single layer. Sear evenly on all sides, tossing occasionally, until cooked through or no longer pink and golden brown on the edges, about 7 minutes. Use a slotted spoon to transfer the cooked chicken to a plate. Repeat until all the chicken is cooked.

Add the ghee to the pan. When it melts, toss in the onion, mushrooms, zucchini, and carrots. Cook, stirring occasionally, until the vegetables are just cooked and slightly tender (you don't want them too soft—I like a little crunch to mine), about 4 minutes. Return the cooked chicken to the skillet and add the toasted sesame seeds. Cook, stirring, for 2 more minutes. Transfer the mixture to a plate and serve with the magic mustard sauce.

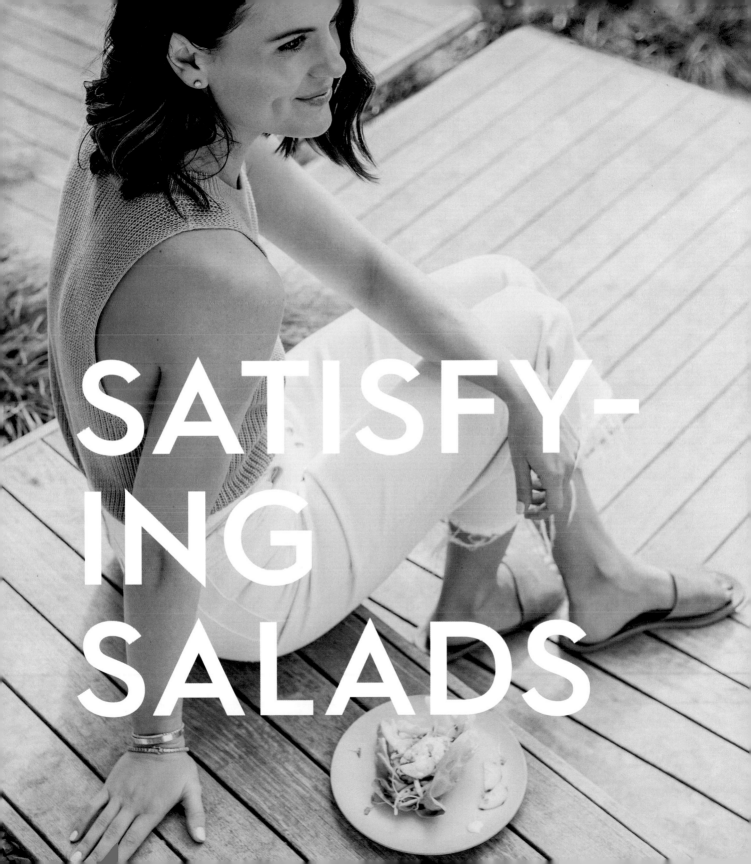

SATISFY-ING SALADS

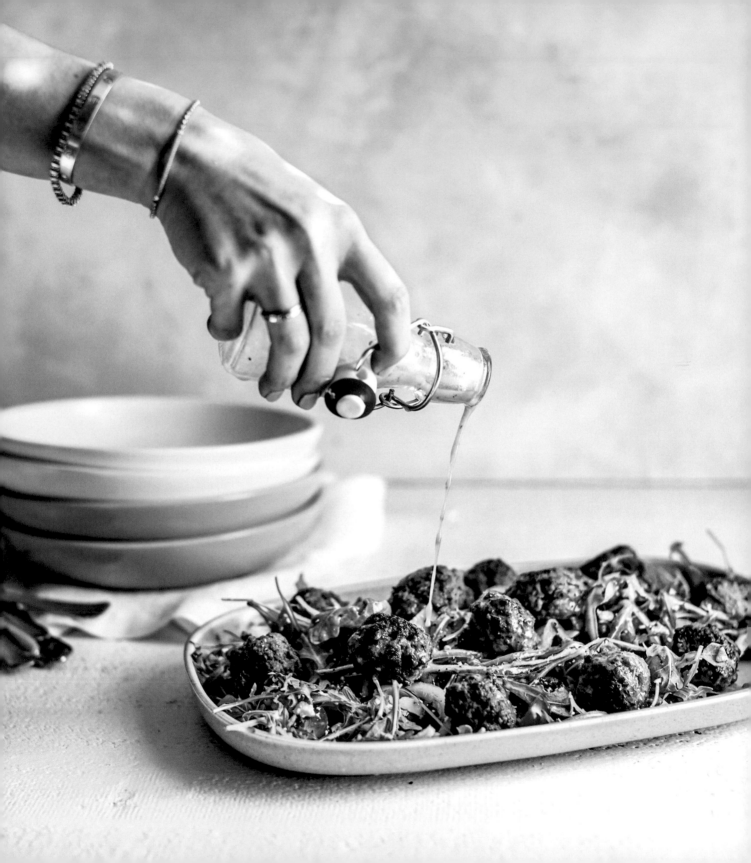

GREEK SALAD *with* LAMB MEATBALLS

SERVES 4
➔ GLUTEN-FREE
➔ DAIRY-FREE IF MODIFIED
➔ PALEO IF MODIFIED
➔ WHOLE30 IF MODIFIED
➔ GRAIN-FREE
Total time: 40 MINUTES

These Greek-style lamb meatballs are an absolute staple in our house. I absolutely love their deep, rich flavor, in addition to the fact that they can be served in so many ways. For busy weeknights, I serve them alongside a nourishing and satisfying Greek-style salad. Other fun ways we serve the meatballs are over a rice pilaf, stuffed in a pita pocket, or even over some gluten-free pasta. If you love Mediterranean food, you gotta make this one and dig into all of the glorious flavors!

MAKE THE GREEK DRESSING In a small jar or container with a fitted lid, combine the olive oil, red wine vinegar, lemon juice, mustard, oregano, salt, and pepper. Cover, then shake vigorously until well combined. Set aside.

MAKE THE SALAD In a large bowl, combine the arugula, cucumbers, cherry tomatoes, olives, red onion, and feta, if using. Do not toss yet. Set aside.

MAKE THE LAMB MEATBALLS Line a large plate with parchment paper and set aside. In a large bowl, combine the lamb, egg yolk, mint, parsley, garlic, mustard, salt, pepper, oregano, and red pepper flakes. Use your hands to mix until just combined. Using a tablespoon or small scoop, form the meat into 1-inch round balls. Transfer to the parchment-lined plate.

Heat the oil in a large skillet over medium-high heat. Swirl the pan to coat the bottom of the skillet evenly and carefully add the meatballs in a single layer. Fry the meatballs until they are

{ continued }

FOR THE GREEK DRESSING

- ¼ cup extra virgin olive oil
- 2 tablespoons red wine vinegar
- 1 tablespoon fresh lemon juice (½ lemon)
- 2 teaspoons Dijon mustard
- 1 teaspoon dried oregano
- ½ teaspoon kosher salt
- ¼ teaspoon freshly ground black pepper

FOR THE SALAD

- 4 cups packed baby arugula
- 1 large cucumber, quartered lengthwise and sliced into ¼-inch pieces (2 cups)
- 1½ cups halved cherry tomatoes
- ½ cup Kalamata olives, pitted and halved
- ½ medium red onion, thinly sliced (1 cup)
- 4 ounces crumbled feta cheese (omit for dairy-free, paleo, Whole30)

FOR THE LAMB MEATBALLS
(on following page)

FOR THE LAMB MEATBALLS

1½ pounds ground lamb (or 80 percent lean ground beef)

1 large egg yolk

1 tablespoon finely chopped fresh mint leaves

1 tablespoon finely chopped fresh flat-leaf parsley leaves

2 garlic cloves, minced

1 teaspoon Dijon mustard

1 teaspoon kosher salt

½ teaspoon freshly ground black pepper

½ teaspoon dried oregano

¼ teaspoon crushed red pepper flakes

1 tablespoon extra virgin olive oil, for frying

browned on all sides and cooked through (or no longer pink in the center), 2 to 3 minutes per side. Transfer the cooked meatballs to a paper towel–lined plate.

TO ASSEMBLE Drizzle your desired amount of dressing onto the salad and gently toss to evenly coat. Serve the dressed salad with the lamb meatballs and enjoy.

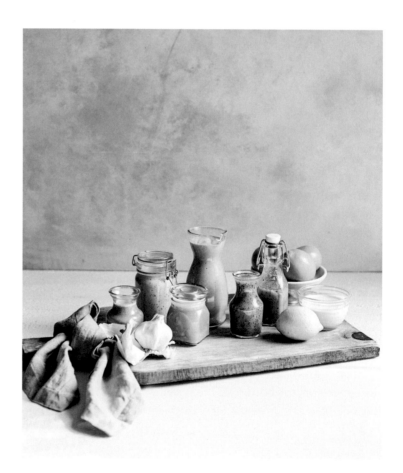

SALMON POKE *and* KALE SALAD BOWLS

SERVES 6

→ GLUTEN-FREE
→ DAIRY-FREE
→ PALEO IF MODIFIED
→ WHOLE30 IF MODIFIED
→ GRAIN-FREE IF MODIFIED

Total time: 30 MINUTES
(BUT DON'T FORGET TO
MARINATE YOUR POKE FIRST!)

This is the dish to make when the sun is shining, and you have friends and family over for a laid-back day of hanging outdoors. It's a summer staple at our house because it's fresh, fast, and healthy. Your guests don't need to know how easy it really is to make poke. So the next time you're hosting a warm-weather get-together, seriously impress them with this recipe!

MAKE THE POKE In a large bowl, combine the salmon, green onions, sesame oil, coconut aminos, avocado oil, jalapeño, black and white sesame seeds, and salt. Using a spoon, gently toss until just combined. Cover with plastic wrap and refrigerate to allow the salmon to marinate for at least 30 minutes or up to 2 hours.

MAKE THE KALE SALAD Rinse the kale and pat it dry. Fold each kale leaf in half, lengthwise, then cut away and discard the ribs. Next, working in batches of several leaves, roll up the leaves like a cigar and slice them into thin ribbons.

Add the kale to a large bowl. Drizzle with the avocado oil and coconut aminos and season with kosher salt. With your hands, gently massage the kale (similar to how you would knead dough) for 3 to 5 minutes, until the kale has softened and wilted slightly.

{ continued }

FOR THE POKE

2 pounds sushi-grade salmon or tuna, cut into ½-inch cubes (see Note)

3 large green onions (white and green parts), thinly sliced

3 tablespoons toasted sesame oil

3 tablespoons coconut aminos

3 tablespoons avocado oil

1 small jalapeño, seeded and finely diced

2 teaspoons black sesame seeds

2 teaspoons white sesame seeds

1 teaspoon kosher salt

FOR THE KALE

1 bunch green kale

3 tablespoons avocado oil

3 tablespoons coconut aminos

½ teaspoon kosher salt, or more to taste

TO ASSEMBLE
(on following page)

TO ASSEMBLE

- 2 avocados, cubed
- 2 tablespoons fresh lime juice (1 lime)
- 3 cups sushi rice, cooked according to the package directions (omit for Whole30, paleo, and grain-free)
- 1 medium English cucumber, thinly sliced
- 1 cup macadamia nuts, roughly chopped

  Lime wedges

  Black sesame seeds

TO ASSEMBLE Remove the poke from the fridge and add the cubed avocado and lime juice. Gently toss once more to combine.

Divide the rice (if using), kale, poke, and sliced cucumber among six bowls. Garnish with the chopped macadamia nuts, lime wedges, and an extra sprinkle of black sesame seeds.

from
MY KITCHEN
to YOURS

Where can you find sushi-grade fish? If you don't have a good seafood market that offers it, try checking in the freezer section of your grocery store.

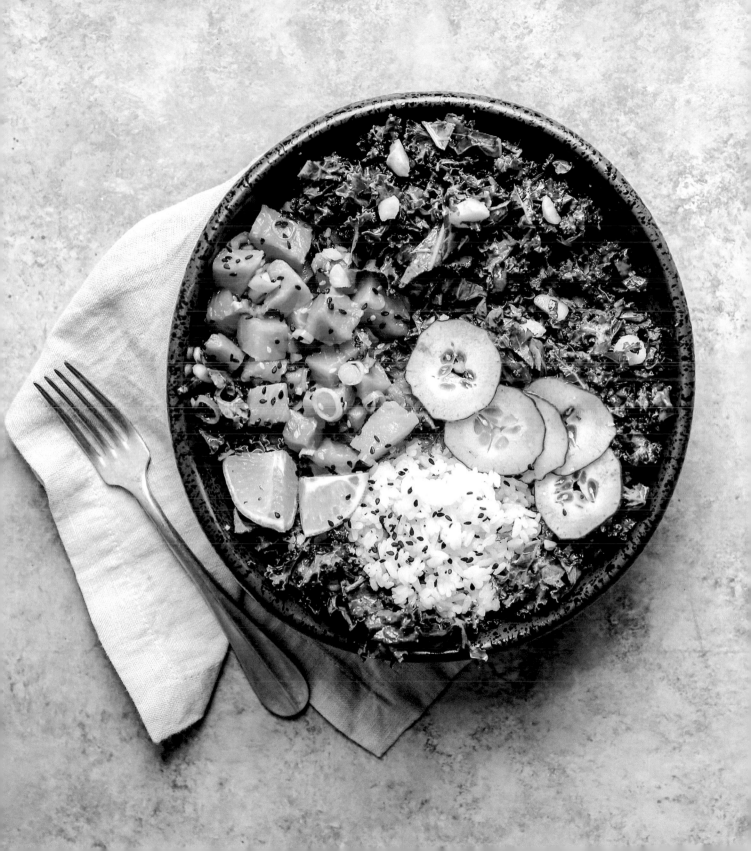

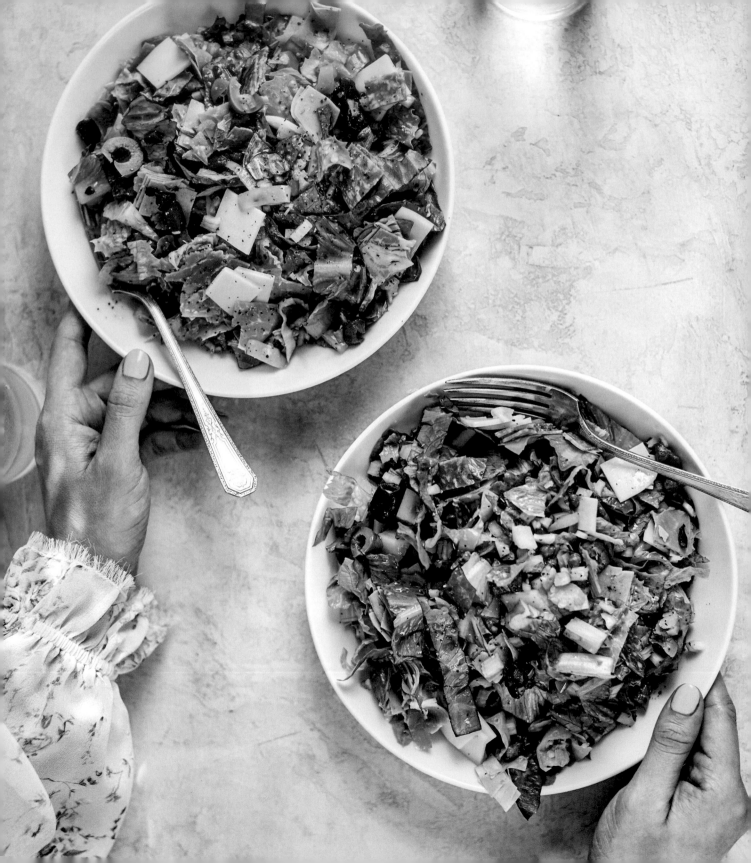

CHOPPED MUFFULETTA SALAD

SERVES 4

→ GLUTEN-FREE

→ DAIRY-FREE IF MODIFIED

→ GRAIN-FREE

Total time: 30 MINUTES

One of my secret powers is my ability to transform my favorite sandwiches into hearty and delicious salads. A "sandwich salad," as we like to call it in our home. The muffuletta as silly as it sounds, is a top-notch sandwich that originated in New Orleans. Layers of various meats are piled high on thick, soft bread and my favorite part? The olive salad that gives the muffuletta its special flavor.

This salad rendition of the muffuletta is perfect for a night you don't want to fire up the kitchen and instead have a "no cook" meal. Spending just a little time chopping and tossing, you'll have dinner on the table in no time and an unforgettable salad!

In a small jar, combine the dressing ingredients and shake until well combined.

Place all of the salad ingredients in a very large salad bowl. Drizzle desired amount of dressing over the salad and toss to coat evenly. Serve immediately.

FOR THE DRESSING

- ¼ cup extra virgin olive oil
- ¼ cup red wine vinegar
- 1 teaspoon Dijon mustard
- ½ teaspoon kosher salt
- ½ teaspoon freshly ground black pepper

FOR THE SALAD

- 8 cups chopped romaine lettuce (2 medium-size heads of lettuce)
- 1 cup loosely chopped pitted olives (preferably mixed olives)
- 2 tablespoons capers, drained
- ½ cup jarred roasted red bell peppers, drained and chopped
- ½ cup jarred peperoncini, drained and chopped
- ½ cup finely diced shallots (2 large)
- ½ cup finely chopped celery (2 stalks)
- 4 ounces thinly sliced mortadella, cut into ½-inch dice (can substitute ham)
- 3 ounces sliced genoa salami, cut into ½-inch dice
- 1½ ounces thinly sliced capicola, cut into ½-inch dice (can substitute spicy salami)
- 3½ ounces sliced provolone cheese, cut into ½-inch dice (optional, omit if dairy-free)

SERVES 3

→ GLUTEN-FREE

→ DAIRY-FREE

→ PALEO

→ WHOLE30

→ GRAIN-FREE

Total time: 35 MINUTES

HAMBURGER SALAD *with* CREAMY JALAPEÑO DRESSING

Over the years of living a mostly gluten-free, grain-free lifestyle, I've come to appreciate that a bun-less burger is a super simple and satisfying weeknight meal. You still get the big juicy burger and all the fixings, just no bun. Don't get me wrong, I do miss the bun on occasion, but when you dress a burger with this creamy jalapeño dressing and make a big salad out of the affair, it certainly makes up for it.

FOR THE CREAMY JALAPEÑO DRESSING

- ¾ cup homemade mayo (page 281)
- ½ cup fresh cilantro leaves
- 2 small jalapeños, seeded and roughly chopped (⅓ cup)
- 2 garlic cloves
- 2 tablespoons red wine vinegar
- 1 teaspoon kosher salt
- ½ teaspoon freshly ground black pepper

FOR THE HAMBURGERS

- 1 pound ground beef, 80 percent lean
  Kosher salt
  Freshly ground black pepper
- 2 tablespoons extra-virgin olive oil

TO ASSEMBLE

- 4 cups chopped romaine lettuce (1 large head)
- ½ medium red onion, thinly sliced (1 cup)
- 1 large tomato, sliced
- 1 avocado, sliced

MAKE THE CREAMY JALAPEÑO DRESSING In a food processor or blender, combine the mayo, cilantro, jalapeños, garlic, vinegar, salt, and pepper and blend until smooth. Set aside.

MAKE THE HAMBURGERS Using your hands, form the ground beef (try not to overwork the meat) into 3 even hamburger patties. Season the patties on both sides generously with salt and pepper.

Heat the oil in a cast-iron skillet over medium-high heat, or brush the oil over the grates of a grill over medium-high heat. Cook the burgers for 3 to 4 minutes per side, until you've reached your desired doneness. (I do mine for 3 minutes per side for medium.)

TO ASSEMBLE Divide the lettuce, onion, tomato, and avocado between 3 bowls. Top each salad with a hamburger patty and drizzle with your desired amount of creamy jalapeño dressing.

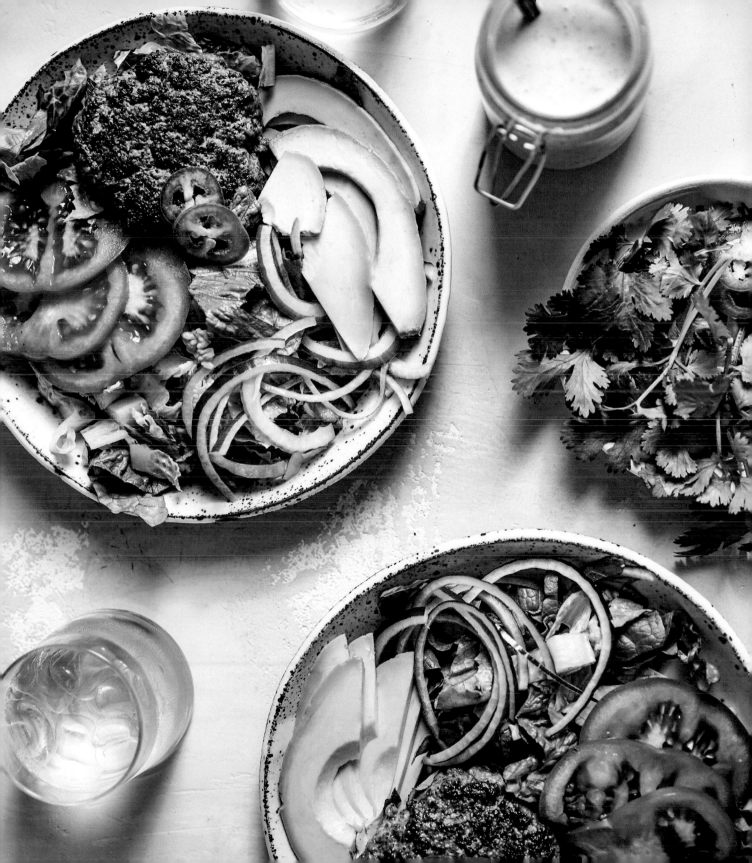

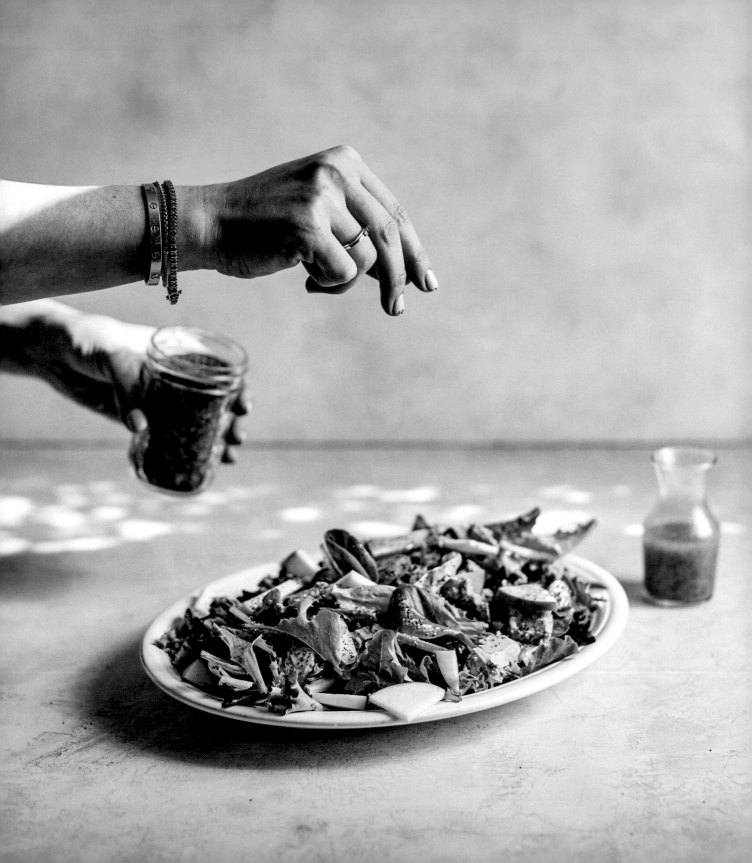

SIMPLE WALDORF TUNA SALAD

SERVES 2

→ GLUTEN-FREE

→ DAIRY-FREE

→ PALEO

→ WHOLE30 IF MODIFIED

→ GRAIN-FREE

Total time: 15 MINUTES

If there were a contest for easiest recipe in this book, this one takes the cake. And it's one of my go-to recipes to make because, let's be honest, there are always those nights when cooking just isn't in the cards. So instead of ordering takeout, try whipping up this simple salad instead. It has layers of great flavors and textures, including a slightly sweet and creamy poppy seed dressing, and comes together in 15 minutes or less.

MAKE THE POPPY SEED DRESSING In a small bowl, whisk together the olive oil, lemon juice, honey, Dijon, poppy seeds, salt, and pepper. Taste and adjust the seasoning with more salt and pepper, if desired. Set aside.

MAKE THE SALAD In a large bowl, combine the greens, grapes, apples, and walnuts. Drizzle with your desired amount of dressing and toss until everything is evenly coated. Add the tuna and give the salad one final gentle toss.

FOR THE POPPY SEED DRESSING

- 2 tablespoons extra virgin olive oil
- 2 tablespoons fresh lemon juice (1 lemon)
- 1 tablespoon honey (omit for Whole30)
- 1 teaspoon mustard
- ½ teaspoon poppy seeds
- ½ teaspoon kosher salt
- ¼ teaspoon freshly ground black pepper

FOR THE SALAD

- 4 cups packed mixed greens
- 1 cup halved red seedless grapes
- 1 cup thinly sliced red apple, cut into 1-inch pieces (1 medium)
- 1 cup walnuts, roughly chopped
- 2 (5-ounce) cans of tuna, drained and broken into bite-size pieces

SERVES 2

→ GLUTEN-FREE

→ DAIRY-FREE

→ PALEO

→ WHOLE30

→ GRAIN-FREE

Total time: 35 MINUTES

STEAK HOUSE CAESAR SALAD

FOR THE CAESAR DRESSING

- 1 cup homemade mayo (page 281)
- 2 tablespoons fresh lemon juice (1 lemon)
- 4 anchovy fillets in olive oil, or 2 teaspoons anchovy paste
- 3 garlic cloves
- 2 teaspoons Dijon mustard
- 1 tablespoon red wine vinegar
- ½ teaspoon kosher salt
- ¼ teaspoon freshly ground black pepper

FOR THE STEAK AND SHRIMP

- 1 pound filet mignon, sirloin steak, or hanger steak
- ½ pound peeled, deveined, tail-on jumbo shrimp
- ½ teaspoon kosher salt
- ½ teaspoon freshly ground black pepper
- 2 tablespoons avocado oil (or other high-heat oil)
- 1 medium head of romaine lettuce, quartered lengthwise

I call this salad my "steak house special" because it combines everything I love about dining out at an old-school steak house: a wedge or Caesar salad to start, plus surf 'n' turf for my main course. In this recipe, I drizzle a Caesar-style dressing over a wedge of romaine lettuce and serve it alongside a juicy steak and seared shrimp. It's an easy-to-make meal with lots of gratification, especially when you scale up to entertain guests.

MAKE THE CAESAR DRESSING In a food processor or blender, combine the mayo, lemon juice, anchovies, garlic, mustard, red wine vinegar, salt, and pepper. Blend until smooth and season with more salt and pepper to taste, if desired. Cover and refrigerate until ready to use (see Note).

MAKE THE STEAK AND SHRIMP Using paper towels, pat dry both the steak and shrimp. Season both sides of the steaks generously with salt and pepper.

Heat the oil in a cast-iron skillet over high heat until it begins to smoke lightly. Using tongs, carefully place the steak in the skillet. Cook until a deep brown crust forms, 3 to 4 minutes per side for medium-rare or 5 to 6 minutes for medium-well. Transfer the steak to a cutting board and let it rest for 8 to 10 minutes to allow the juices to settle back into the meat.

Reduce the heat to medium and add the shrimp to the skillet. Cook until pink, about 2 minutes per side. Remove the shrimp from the pan and set aside.

{ continued }

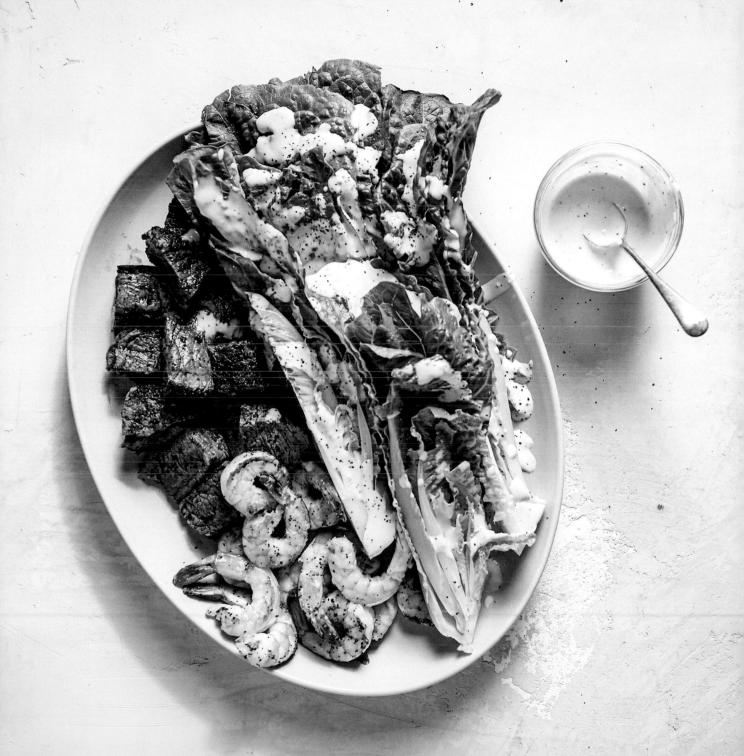

ASSEMBLE THE SALAD Divide the romaine wedges between 2 plates and drizzle with your desired amount of Caesar dressing. Plate the steak and shrimp alongside. Serve and enjoy!

from
MY KITCHEN
to YOURS

This Caesar dressing is great to make for meal prep and use all week long. It keeps for about 5 days in the refrigerator.

BUN CHA

SERVES 4
→ GLUTEN-FREE
→ DAIRY-FREE
→ PALEO IF MODIFIED
→ GRAIN-FREE IF MODIFIED
Total time: 40 MINUTES

Vietnamese Spicy Pork Meatballs with Fresh Noodle Salad

One of my all-time favorite restaurants is Elizabeth Street Cafe in Austin, Texas. Anytime I'm visiting, it's always on the top of my to-do list as far as eats go. They make an incredible marinated pork bun that I order every time I go, which I realized I could re-create at home—with my own healthier spin, of course. Since pork can easily dry out when grilled, I decided it'd be best to do pork meatballs instead. Best decision I've ever made! These pork meatballs are everything I have ever dreamed of in meatball form—a little spicy, a little tangy, a little ginger-y. Plus I serve them with nuoc cham, a Vietnamese dipping sauce that has an irresistible sweet, sour, salty, and spicy flavor. It keeps for up to 4 months in the fridge, so I highly recommend using it to brighten seafood, add a salty tang to beef or pork, or simply spooning it over steamed rice or noodles for an easy, delicious dinner.

This dish has quickly become one of my husband's most-requested and is one of my personal favorites, too.

MAKE THE NUOC CHAM SAUCE In a medium bowl, combine ⅔ cup water with the fish sauce, lime juice, coconut sugar, rice vinegar, chiles, and garlic. Whisk until the sugar has dissolved. Set aside.

MAKE THE PORK MEATBALLS In a large bowl, combine the pork, shallot, garlic, chiles, fish sauce, coconut aminos, ginger, salt, and pepper. Use your hands to mix until just combined.

{ continued }

FOR THE NUOC CHAM SAUCE

- ⅓ cup fish sauce (I use Red Boat)
- ¼ cup fresh lime juice (about 2 limes)
- 3 tablespoons coconut palm sugar
- 2 tablespoons rice vinegar
- 1 to 3 bird's eye chiles, very thinly sliced (1 for mild, 3 for hot)
- 2 garlic cloves, minced

FOR THE PORK MEATBALLS

- 2 pounds ground pork
- 1 medium shallot, minced (3 tablespoons)
- 3 garlic cloves, minced
- 2 bird's eye chiles, very thinly sliced
- 1 tablespoon fish sauce (I use Red Boat)
- 2 tablespoons coconut aminos
- 1 (½-inch) piece fresh ginger, finely grated
- ½ teaspoon kosher salt
- ¼ teaspoon freshly ground black pepper
- 2 tablespoons extra virgin olive or avocado oil, for frying

TO ASSEMBLE
(on following page)

TO ASSEMBLE

- 4 cups mixed spring greens
- 2 small carrots, cut into matchsticks
- 1 medium English cucumber, seeded and thinly sliced into matchsticks
- 1½ cups bean sprouts
- ¼ cup fresh mint leaves
- ¼ cup fresh Thai or regular basil leaves
- ¼ cup fresh cilantro leaves
- 8 ounces rice vermicelli noodles, cooked according to package directions (replace with daikon radish if paleo or grain-free)
- Lime wedges
- 1 cup cashews, roughly chopped

Scoop 2 tablespoons of the meatball mixture at a time onto a parchment-lined plate and use your hands to form each into a ball. Repeat until you've used all the meat.

In a large nonstick skillet over medium-high, heat the oil. Working in batches so you don't crowd the pan, add the meatballs and arrange them in a single layer. Fry them on all sides until golden brown, about 2 minutes per side. Reduce the heat to medium-low and continue to cook until the meatballs are cooked through or no longer pink, 4 to 6 minutes more. Transfer the meatballs to a paper towel–lined plate.

TO ASSEMBLE Divide the spring greens, carrots, cucumber, bean sprouts, mint, basil, and cilantro among four bowls. Add the meatballs and ½ cup of the cooked noodles to each bowl (if using). Spoon your desired amount of nuoc cham sauce over the bowls, add the lime wedges, and sprinkle with the chopped cashews.

from
MY KITCHEN
to YOURS

My kiddos love this dish. To keep it mild enough for their taste buds, though, I only use one bird's eye chile in both the meat and the sauce when I serve this to them.

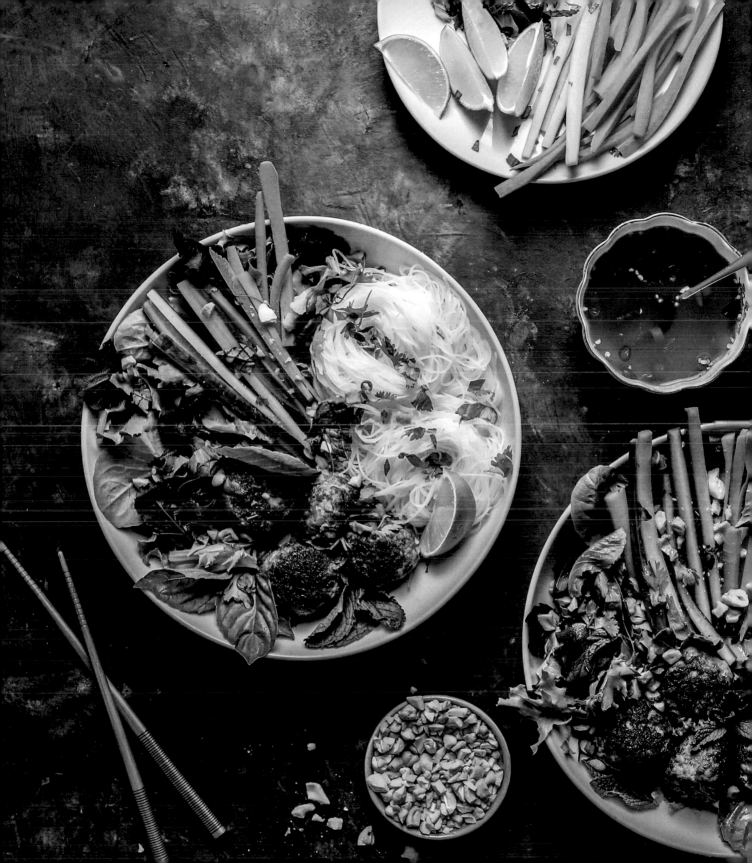

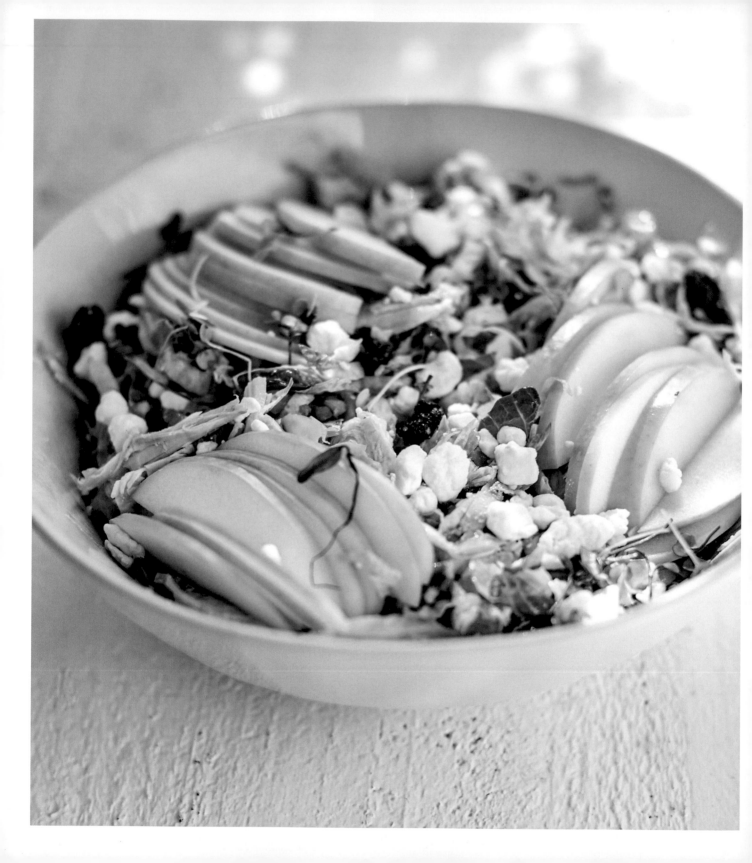

BRUSSELS SPROUT SALAD *with* HONEY-MUSTARD VINAIGRETTE

SERVES 4

→ GLUTEN-FREE

→ DAIRY-FREE IF MODIFIED

→ PALEO IF MODIFIED

→ GRAIN-FREE

Total time: 20 MINUTES

It's no secret that Brussels sprouts are really good for you. But if you're looking to get your veggies in and actually enjoy the taste—this recipe is perfect for you! It's delicious, nutritious, and easy to make. My favorite part is that the shredded Brussels sprouts are sturdy enough to keep well after they are already dressed. In fact, it's one of those salads that actually gets better with time, making it perfect for meal prep!

Combine all of the dressing ingredients in a jar and shake until well combined. Set aside.

Place the shaved Brussels sprouts, arugula, shredded chicken, sliced apple, dried cranberries, chopped walnuts, and goat cheese (if using) in a large serving bowl.

Pour the dressing over the salad and toss to coat evenly. Let rest at room temp for about 10 minutes before serving (this helps marinate the Brussels sprouts a bit).

FOR THE DRESSING

- ¼ cup extra virgin olive oil
- 2 teaspoons Dijon mustard
- 2 tablespoons apple cider vinegar
- 2 tablespoons fresh lemon juice (1 lemon)
- 2 tablespoons honey
- 2 cloves garlic, minced
- 1 teaspoon kosher salt
- ½ teaspoon freshly ground black pepper

FOR THE SALAD

- 12 ounces Brussels sprouts, shaved (about 4 cups; see Note)
- 2 cups baby arugula
- 3 cups shredded chicken (rotisserie or see page 279)
- 1½ cups thinly sliced Granny Smith apple (1 medium apple)
- 1 cup dried, unsweetened cranberries
- 1 cup loosely chopped walnuts
- 4 ounces crumbled goat cheese (omit for paleo and dairy-free)

from
MY KITCHEN
to YOURS

You can buy Brussels sprouts already shaved at some grocery stores. If you can't find them, here is how to "shave" them: First, cut off the woody ends of the Brussels sprouts and discard any discolored outer leaves. Then, carefully shred them with a sharp knife by slicing them as thinly as possible. It's a bit of a hand workout, but worth it!

SERVES 4

→ GLUTEN-FREE

→ DAIRY-FREE

→ PALEO

→ WHOLE30

→ GRAIN-FREE

Total time: 30 MINUTES

KALE *and* MINT SALAD *with* "PEANUT" VINAIGRETTE

FOR THE "PEANUT" VINAIGRETTE

- 2 tablespoons rice vinegar
- 2 tablespoons unsweetened, creamy cashew butter (or any creamy nut butter of your choice)
- 2 tablespoons coconut aminos
- 1 tablespoon fresh lime juice (½ lime)
- 1 garlic clove
- 1 (½-inch) piece fresh ginger, finely grated
- 1 teaspoon toasted sesame oil
- 1 teaspoon chili oil or ¼ teaspoon crushed red pepper flakes (optional)
- Kosher salt and freshly ground black pepper

FOR THE SALAD

- 1 bunch green kale
- 2 cups shredded chicken (rotisserie or see page 279)
- ½ cup cashews, loosely chopped
- ¼ cup fresh mint leaves, chopped
- 1 tablespoon toasted sesame seeds

This is the salad of all salads—it turns kale haters into kale lovers, and the dressing is so good you might as well pour it in a cocktail glass and drink it. It's satisfying, easy to make, and absolutely delicious! To make this vegetarian, simply omit the shredded chicken.

MAKE THE "PEANUT" VINAIGRETTE In a food processor or blender, combine the rice vinegar, cashew butter, coconut aminos, lime juice, garlic, ginger, toasted sesame oil, chili oil, salt, and pepper. Blend until smooth. Set aside.

MAKE THE SALAD Rinse the kale and pat it dry. Fold each kale leaf in half, then cut away and discard the ribs. Next, working in batches of several leaves, roll up the leaves like a cigar and slice them into thin ribbons. Place the kale in a large bowl and toss with the shredded chicken, cashews, mint, and sesame seeds. Drizzle with the vinaigrette and toss consistently until the kale is very well coated and starting to wilt, 3 to 5 minutes.

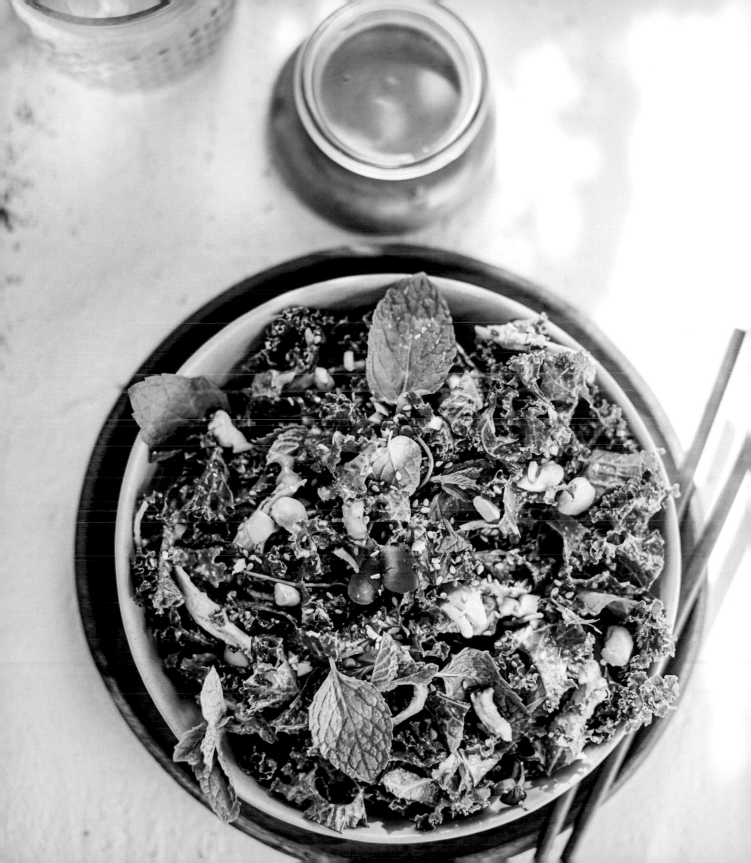

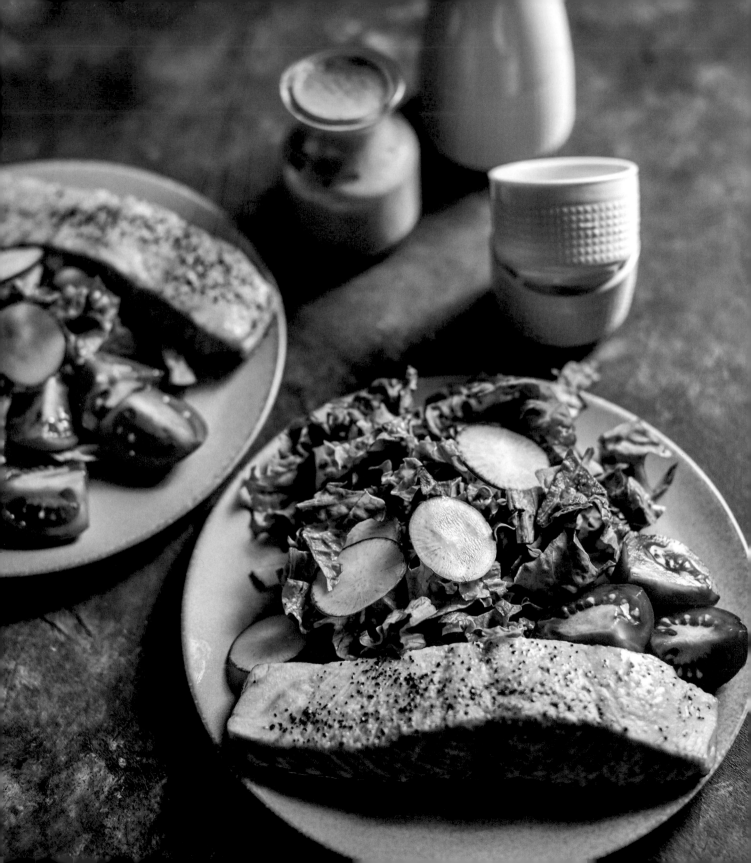

CARROT-GINGER SALAD *with* BAKED SALMON

SERVES 4
→ GLUTEN-FREE
→ DAIRY-FREE
→ PALEO
→ WHOLE30
→ GRAIN-FREE
Total Cook Time: 35 MINUTES

One of my favorite parts about going to a Japanese-style restaurant is the carrot-ginger salad that typically gets served to start the meal. It's so simple—usually just a bed of iceberg lettuce, maybe some shredded veggies thrown in too—but the dressing does all the talking. It's light, refreshing, and yet surprisingly creamy. It's also impossibly easy to make at home—all you need is a high-powered blender that can break down the carrots and fresh ginger—and you'll end up with a versatile dressing that will make just about any weeknight meal an exciting one. I especially love tossing it with bright, fresh veggies like tomatoes and radishes and tufting it all beside simple baked salmon.

MAKE THE SALMON Preheat the oven to 375°F. Line a large baking sheet with parchment paper.

Arrange the salmon fillets on the prepared baking sheet. Drizzle each with 1 teaspoon olive oil and brush to fully coat the top of the fillets. Sprinkle with salt and pepper and bake for 15 to 20 minutes, until the salmon flakes easily with a fork. Set aside and let cool slightly.

MAKE THE CARROT-GINGER DRESSING In a high-powered blender, combine the carrots, shallot, and ginger and process until very finely chopped. Add the olive oil, coconut aminos, rice vinegar, sesame oil, fish sauce, salt, pepper, and 1 tablespoon water. Blend on high until very smooth. Add more salt and pepper

{ continued }

FOR THE SALMON

- 4 (6- to 8-ounce) center-cut salmon fillets
- 4 teaspoons extra virgin olive oil
- Kosher salt and freshly ground black pepper

FOR THE CARROT-GINGER DRESSING

- 2 large carrots, roughly chopped (1½ cups)
- ¼ cup finely diced shallots (1 large)
- 1 (1½ inch) piece fresh ginger, roughly chopped (about 2 tablespoons)
- ½ cup extra virgin olive oil
- ¼ cup coconut aminos
- 2 tablespoons rice vinegar
- 1 tablespoon plus 1 teaspoon toasted sesame oil
- 1 tablespoon fish sauce (I use Red Boat)
- ½ teaspoon kosher salt
- ¼ teaspoon freshly ground black pepper

FOR THE SALAD
(on following page)

FOR THE SALAD

1 head green leaf lettuce, ends trimmed and leaves chopped into bite-size pieces

4 Campari tomatoes, quartered

4 radishes, thinly sliced

to taste if necessary. You can make the dressing ahead and store it in the fridge for 5 to 7 days.

ASSEMBLE THE SALAD In a large bowl, toss together the lettuce, tomatoes, and radishes. Drizzle with desired amount of dressing and give another toss. Divide between 4 plates and serve each with a salmon fillet.

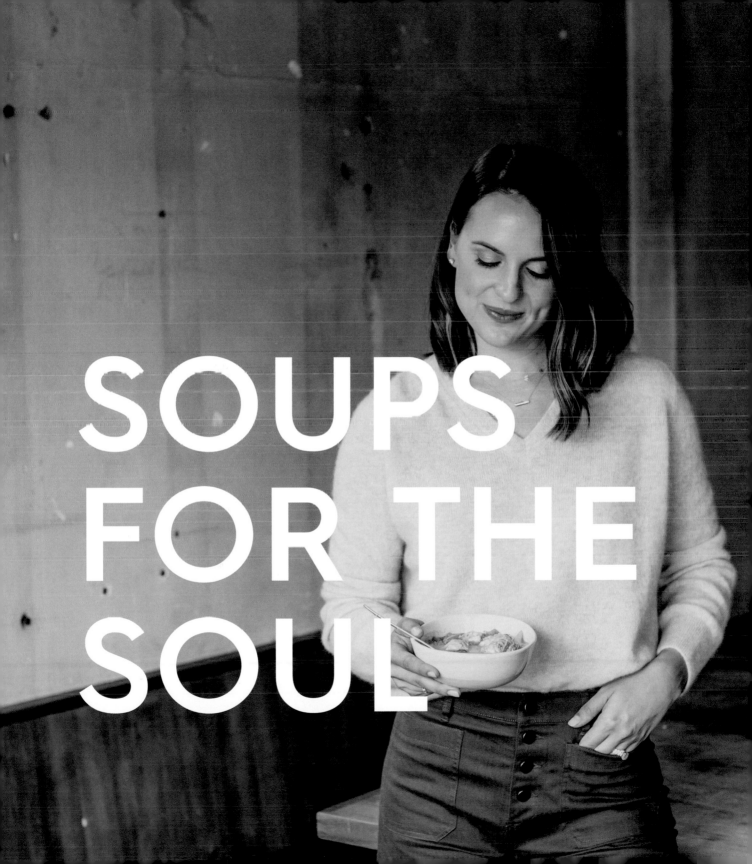

SOUPS FOR THE SOUL

SERVES 4

→ GLUTEN-FREE

→ DAIRY-FREE

→ PALEO

→ WHOLE30

→ GRAIN-FREE

Total time: 30 MINUTES

CREAMY TORTILLA-LESS SOUP

2 tablespoons extra virgin olive oil

2 cups diced yellow onion (2 medium)

4 cloves garlic, minced

1 tablespoon seeded and diced jalapeño (½ medium)

½ teaspoon kosher salt, or more to taste

¼ teaspoon freshly ground black pepper, or more to taste

1 tablespoon ground cumin

1 teaspoon ground coriander

1 tablespoon tomato paste

4 cups low-sodium chicken broth

3 cups strained tomatoes (I use Pomi brand)

1 cup jarred, canned, or frozen roasted mild green chiles

1 bay leaf

¼ cup unsweetened full-fat coconut milk

TO ASSEMBLE

2 cups shredded chicken (rotisserie or see page 279)

1 avocado, sliced

¼ cup fresh cilantro leaves

3 radishes, thinly sliced

1 lime, cut into wedges

Growing up in Dallas, one of my most favorite special occasion restaurants is The Mansion at Turtle Creek. A Dallas classic, it is absolutely fantastic and is known for its tortilla soup by the famous local chef, Dean Fearing. I could eat bottomless bowls of that soup all day. Here is my at-home, tortilla-less version of the famous soup. It's a fan favorite on my blog and if you love a creamy soup that packs some heat, make this one to warm you up on a cool night! You'll just love it.

In a Dutch oven or large pot, heat the olive oil over medium heat. Add the onion, garlic, jalapeño, salt, and pepper and cook, stirring, until tender, about 5 minutes.

Add the cumin, coriander, and tomato paste and toast, stirring, until fragrant, 1 to 2 minutes.

Add the broth, strained tomatoes, green chiles, and bay leaf and bring to a boil. Reduce the heat to a simmer and cook, uncovered and stirring occasionally, for 20 minutes for the flavors to meld.

Discard the bay leaf and add the coconut milk. Using an immersion blender or blender, blend soup until very smooth. Taste and add more salt, if desired.

Place ½ cup shredded chicken in the bottom of each bowl. Ladle the soup over. Garnish with avocado slices, cilantro, radishes, and serve with a wedge of lime.

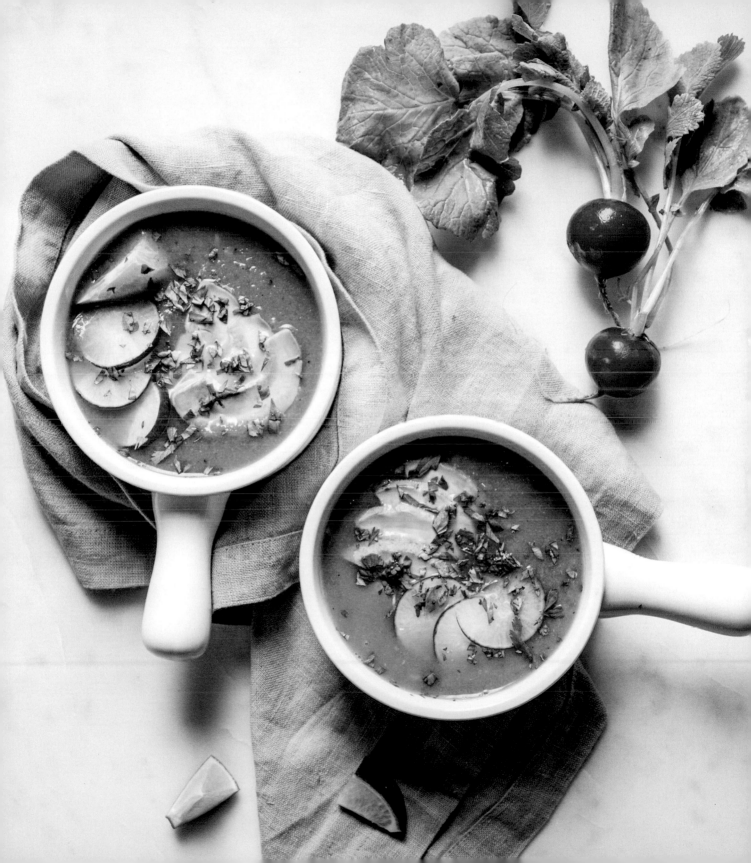

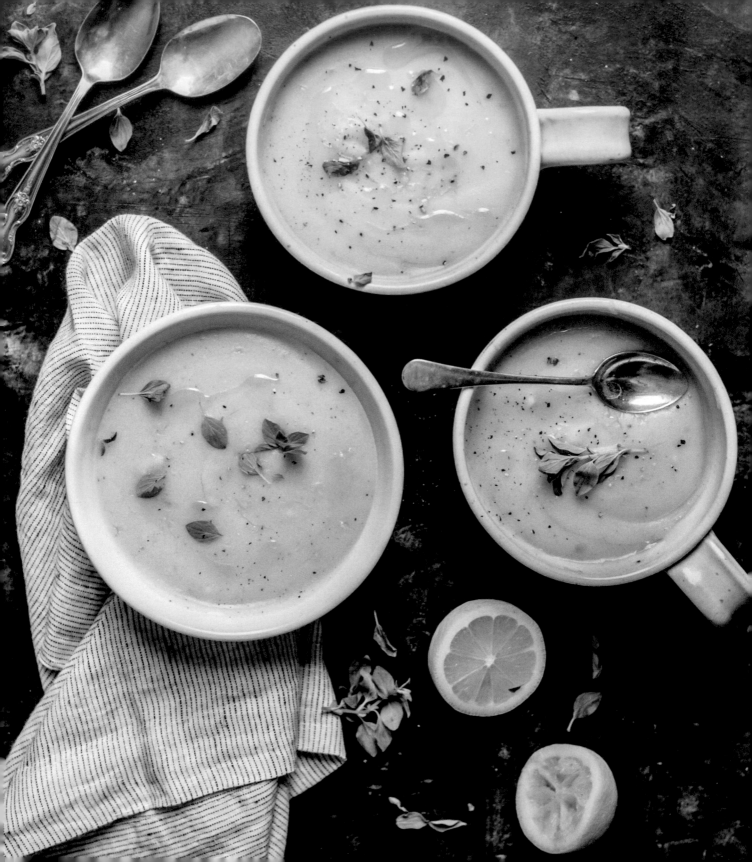

GREEK LEMON *and* OREGANO POTATO SOUP

SERVES 8

→ GLUTEN-FREE

→ DAIRY-FREE

→ PALEO

→ WHOLE30

→ GRAIN-FREE

Total time: 45 MINUTES

One of the dishes I look forward to most when I'm out at a Greek restaurant is roasted Greek potatoes. I crave their bright lemony flavor combined with earthy oregano. I also happen to love a big bowl of creamy potato soup in the winter. So when it came time to dream up the perfect new recipe for colder months, I figured, *Why not combine the two?!* The result is a dish that's a warm, cozy, and satisfying soup with a touch of brightness thanks to the citrus and herbs. It also doesn't hurt that it couldn't be easier to make and is very budget-friendly.

In a Dutch oven or large pot, heat the olive oil over medium heat. Add the onion, garlic, 1 teaspoon of the salt, and pepper. Cook, stirring occasionally, until the onion is tender, 5 to 7 minutes.

Add the potatoes, broth, oregano, and bay leaf and increase the heat to medium-high to bring the soup to a boil. Once boiling, reduce the heat to a simmer, cover, and cook until the potatoes are fork-tender, about 30 minutes.

Remove and discard the bay leaf. Use an immersion blender to blend the soup until creamy and smooth. Alternatively, transfer the soup to a food processor or blender and, working in batches, blend until creamy and smooth then return the soup to the pot.

Gently re-warm the soup over low heat. Stir in the remaining 1 teaspoon of salt plus the lemon juice and cayenne pepper, if using. Allow the flavors to meld, about 5 minutes. Taste the soup and adjust the seasoning with more salt, if desired.

Divide the soup among 8 serving bowls, drizzle with a little olive oil, and garnish with freshly chopped chives or fresh oregano leaves.

- 2 tablespoons extra virgin olive oil, plus more for serving
- 2 cups diced yellow onion (2 medium)
- 4 garlic cloves, finely chopped
- 2 teaspoons kosher salt
- ½ teaspoon freshly ground black pepper
- 2½ pounds (about 5 large) Yukon gold potatoes, peeled and cut into 2-inch cubes
- 4 cups low-sodium chicken or vegetable broth
- 2 teaspoons dried oregano
- 1 bay leaf
- ¼ cup fresh lemon juice (2 lemons)
- ⅛ teaspoon cayenne pepper (optional)
- ¼ cup chopped fresh chives or whole fresh oregano leaves, for serving

SERVES 4
→ GLUTEN-FREE
→ DAIRY-FREE
→ PALEO
→ WHOLE30
→ GRAIN-FREE
Total time: 35 MINUTES

HEALING CHICKEN SOUP

2 tablespoons extra virgin olive oil

½ medium yellow onion, diced (1 cup)

2 celery stalks, roughly chopped (¾ cup)

1 large carrot, roughly chopped (1 cup)

1 teaspoon kosher salt

½ teaspoon freshly ground black pepper

2 garlic cloves, minced

1 (1-inch) piece fresh ginger, finely grated

4 cups low-sodium chicken broth

1½ pounds boneless, skinless chicken breasts

1 sprig fresh rosemary leaves, chopped (1 teaspoon)

3 sprigs fresh thyme leaves (about 1 teaspoon)

½ teaspoon ground turmeric

⅛ teaspoon cayenne pepper (optional)

2 bay leaves

2 cups packed roughly chopped kale (I prefer lacinato)

2 tablespoons fresh lemon juice (1 lemon)

Of all of the folk remedies for when you're feeling under the weather, a bowl of chicken soup is one of the oldest and most reliable. Not only is it soothing, but it also contains healing properties. This recipe in particular is packed with a few extra ingredients that help alleviate cold symptoms, such as anti-inflammatory ginger, turmeric, and garlic. It's also packed with fantastic flavor thanks to the addition of fresh rosemary, thyme, and lemon. Sick or not sick, you'll just love a bowl of this soup for dinner.

In a large pot, heat the olive oil over medium heat. Add the onion, celery, carrot, salt, and pepper and cook, stirring, until the vegetables are tender, 5 to 7 minutes. Add the garlic and ginger and cook, stirring occasionally, for 2 more minutes.

Mix in the broth, chicken, rosemary, thyme, turmeric, cayenne pepper (if using), and bay leaves and bring the soup to a boil. Reduce the heat to a simmer, cover, and cook until the chicken is cooked through and can be easily shredded, about 15 minutes.

Using tongs, transfer the chicken to a cutting board and reduce the heat under the soup to medium. Use two forks to shred chicken into bite-size pieces. Return the shredded chicken to the soup along with the kale and lemon juice. Over medium heat, cook the soup until the kale has just wilted, about 4 more minutes. Remove and discard the bay leaves. Taste the soup and adjust the seasoning with more salt and pepper, if desired.

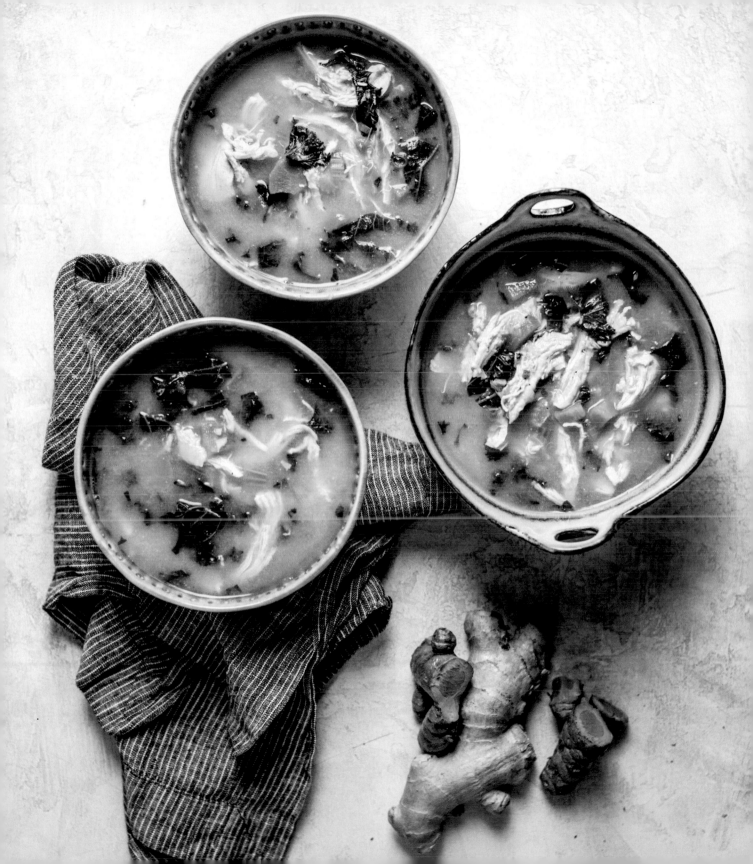

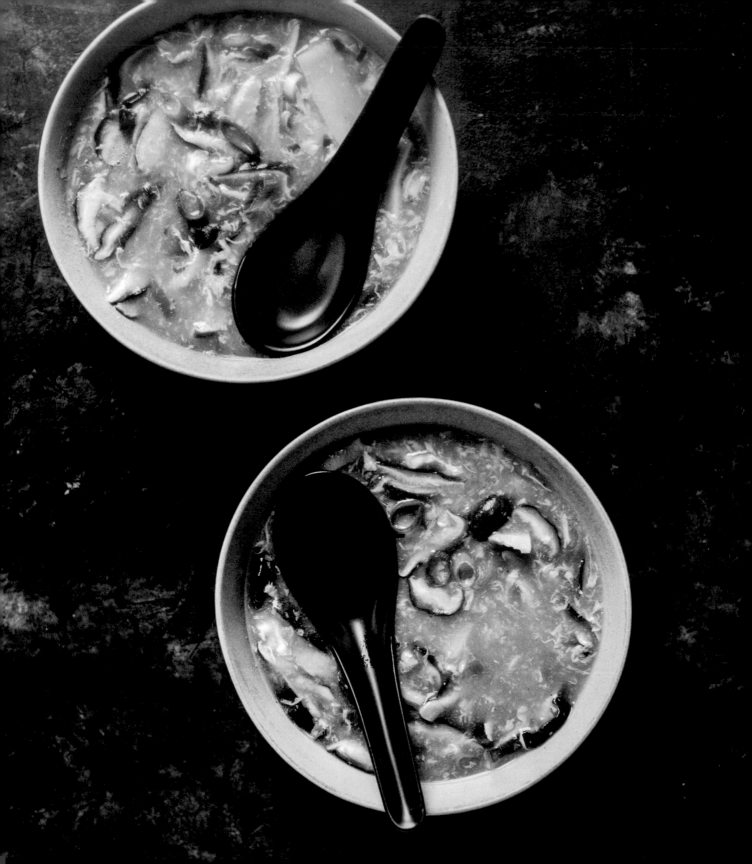

WHOLE30 HOT- and -SOUR SOUP

SERVES 4

→ GLUTEN-FREE

→ DAIRY-FREE

→ PALEO

→ WHOLE30

→ GRAIN-FREE

Total time: 30 MINUTES

Creating a Whole30 rendition of the Chinese classic hot-and-sour soup is like teaching a pig to fly—it seems entirely unlikely. The traditional version is filled with all of the not-so-Whole30-compliant things: soy sauce, cornstarch, sriracha or chili garlic sauce, and tofu, to name a few. But I was on a mission to create a recipe because it's one of my favorite soups ever. This soup is as close as I could possibly get to the real deal—and no matter what, it's absolutely delicious. If you are a hot-and-sour soup lover like me and want to hold the MSG, try this fabulous, clean-eating version in your kitchen!

In a medium bowl, whisk together ½ cup of the chicken broth and the arrowroot until the arrowroot dissolves. Set aside.

In a large skillet, heat the avocado oil over medium heat. Add the ginger, garlic, sesame oil, and red pepper flakes and cook, being careful not to burn, until fragrant, 1 to 2 minutes.

Pour in the remaining 4 cups chicken broth plus the rice vinegar, coconut aminos, fish sauce, and cayenne pepper. Increase the heat to medium-high and bring the mixture to a boil. Once boiling, reduce to a simmer and add the shredded chicken, mushrooms, bamboo shoots (if using), and green onions. Stir in the broth-arrowroot mixture. Cook, stirring occasionally, until the soup has thickened, the mushrooms are cooked through, and the green onions are tender, about 7 minutes.

Reduce the heat to medium-low. While stirring the soup in a circular motion, very slowly drizzle the beaten eggs into the soup in a thin stream to create egg ribbons. Stir in the lime juice and season with salt, if desired. Top with green onions and serve immediately.

4½ cups low-sodium chicken broth

2 tablespoons arrowroot starch

2 tablespoons avocado oil

1 (1½-inch) piece fresh ginger, grated

2 garlic cloves, minced

1 teaspoon toasted sesame oil

¼ teaspoon crushed red pepper flakes

⅓ cup rice vinegar

¼ cup coconut aminos

2 teaspoons fish sauce (I use Red Boat)

⅛ teaspoon cayenne pepper

1½ cups shredded chicken (rotisserie or see page 279)

8 ounces shiitake mushrooms, stemmed and sliced

1 (8-ounce) can bamboo shoots, drained (optional)

2 green onions (white and green parts), thinly sliced, plus more for serving

2 large eggs, beaten

2 tablespoons fresh lime juice (1 lime)

Kosher salt (optional)

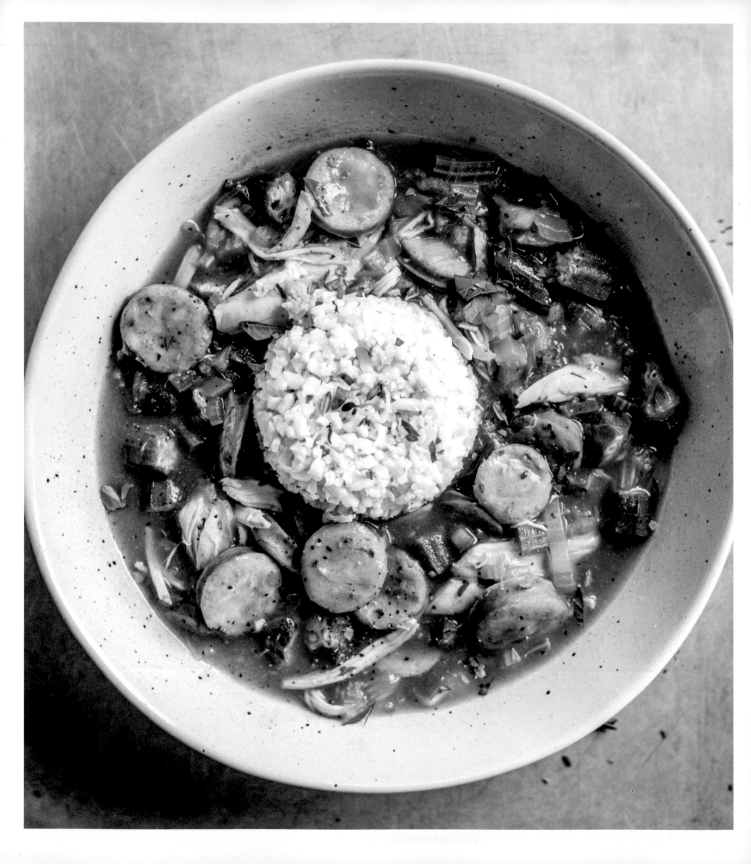

CHICKEN *and* SAUSAGE GUMBO

SERVES 6

→ GLUTEN-FREE

→ DAIRY-FREE

→ PALEO

→ WHOLE30

→ GRAIN-FREE

Total time: 50 MINUTES

Nothing beats a big bowl of gumbo after a long day. It's filling and full of deep, rich flavor that tastes like it's been simmering on the stove all day (though it has decidedly not). This version of the traditional dish is cleaned up and Whole30-compliant, and I also made it a heck of a lot easier to throw together so that you can have it on the dinner table in no time. This recipe is a fan favorite on my blog, but the true stamp of approval comes from my Louisiana friends who tell me how much they love this health-ified version.

Preheat the oven to 425°F.

Line a large baking sheet with parchment paper and spread the okra over the baking sheet. Drizzle with 1 tablespoon oil and toss to evenly coat. Season with a pinch of salt and pepper. Roast until golden brown, 20 to 25 minutes. Set aside.

In a large bowl, combine 1 cup of the broth with the arrowroot. Whisk until the arrowroot has dissolved. Set aside.

In a large pot or Dutch oven, heat the remaining 4 tablespoons oil over medium-high heat. Add the onion, bell pepper, and celery. Season with a pinch of salt and pepper and cook, stirring occasionally, until tender, about 6 minutes. Reduce the heat to medium and add the garlic, tomato paste, cayenne pepper, and thyme. Cook for another 2 minutes. While whisking, slowly add the arrowroot mixture, stirring constantly until well combined and thickened to a gravy-like consistency, about 3 minutes. Once thickened, slowly pour in 3 additional cups of broth, while stirring constantly. Bring the soup to a simmer and let cook, uncovered,

{ continued }

2 cups pre-cut frozen okra

5 tablespoons extra virgin olive or avocado oil

Kosher salt and freshly ground black pepper

5 to 6 cups low-sodium chicken broth

2 tablespoons arrowroot starch

1 cup finely diced yellow onion (½ medium)

1 cup finely diced green bell pepper (½ medium)

¾ cup finely diced celery (3 stalks)

2 garlic cloves, minced

1 tablespoon tomato paste

½ teaspoon cayenne pepper

¼ teaspoon dried thyme

2 cups shredded chicken, (rotisserie or see page 279)

12 ounces cooked no-sugar-added andouille or kielbasa sausage, sliced

2 cups Prepared Cauliflower Rice (page 282), for serving

2 tablespoons chopped fresh flat-leaf parsley leaves, for serving

for 10 minutes to allow the flavors to meld and the soup to thicken a bit more.

Stir in the shredded chicken, andouille sausage, and roasted okra. Add an additional 1 to 2 cups of broth until the gumbo reaches your desired thickness. I like my gumbo a little thinner and soupier, so I do 2 cups. Taste and adjust the seasoning with more salt and pepper if desired. Serve over cauliflower rice. Garnish with parsley.

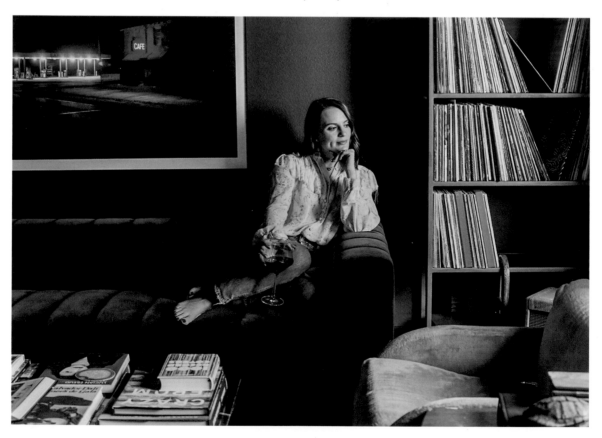

GINGER-SCALLION MEATBALL *and* BOK CHOY SOUP

SERVES 6
→ GLUTEN-FREE
→ DAIRY-FREE
→ PALEO
→ WHOLE30
→ GRAIN-FREE
Total time: 45 MINUTES

Want to know a pro move? Add meatballs to your soup! I am a soup lover through and through; however, my husband and kids are never super-thrilled when soup is on the menu. But when I add meatballs? Very different story. Suddenly a meh dinner is one that everyone is excited about—and without a lot of extra effort. This Asian-inspired soup is my Whole30 ode to wonton soup, where the meatballs have very similar flavor to the garlic-and-ginger-scented filling that's usually inside wontons. Of course, I add some veggies to the broth to make it a well-rounded, wholesome weeknight meal, and that it is! Thanks to the meatballs, it's nice and filling and one the whole family will enjoy.

MAKE THE MEATBALLS Preheat the oven to 350°F. Line two large baking sheets with parchment paper. Set aside.

In a large bowl, combine the ground chicken, almond flour, green onions, egg, garlic, ginger, salt, pepper, sesame oil, and red pepper flakes. Use your hands to mix until just combined.

Using a melon baller or a teaspoon, drop 1- to 1¼-inch balls onto the prepared baking sheets. Use your hands to roll the meatballs into round balls (they don't have to be perfect!). Bake for 30 minutes, or until just cooked through and lightly browned. Set aside.

{ continued }

FOR THE MEATBALLS

- 2 pounds ground chicken thighs (turkey or pork works, too)
- ½ cup almond flour
- 3 large green onions (white and green parts), chopped (¾ cup)
- 1 large egg, lightly beaten
- 2 garlic cloves, minced
- 1 (½-inch) piece fresh ginger, finely grated
- 1 teaspoon kosher salt
- ½ teaspoon freshly ground black pepper
- ½ teaspoon toasted sesame oil
- ½ teaspoon crushed red pepper flakes (optional)

FOR THE SOUP
(on following page)

FOR THE SOUP

2 tablespoons avocado oil

¾ cup diced carrot (1 large)

½ cup diced yellow onion (¼ medium)

Kosher salt and freshly ground black pepper

1½ cups sliced shiitake mushrooms

2 garlic cloves, minced

8 cups low-sodium chicken broth

2 tablespoons coconut aminos

1 teaspoon fish sauce (I use Red Boat)

3 heads baby bok choy, rinsed, ends trimmed, and cut into thirds

2 tablespoons fresh lime juice (1 lime)

MAKE THE SOUP In a Dutch oven or large pot, heat the avocado oil over medium heat. Add the carrot and onion with a pinch each of salt and pepper. Cook until the vegetables are soft and tender, about 5 minutes. Add the mushrooms and garlic and cook for 2 more minutes. Pour in the broth, coconut aminos, and fish sauce and bring to a simmer.

Drop the meatballs and bok choy into the pot and simmer until the book choy is very tender, 8 to 10 more minutes. Add the lime juice and season with salt and pepper to taste. Ladle into bowls and serve!

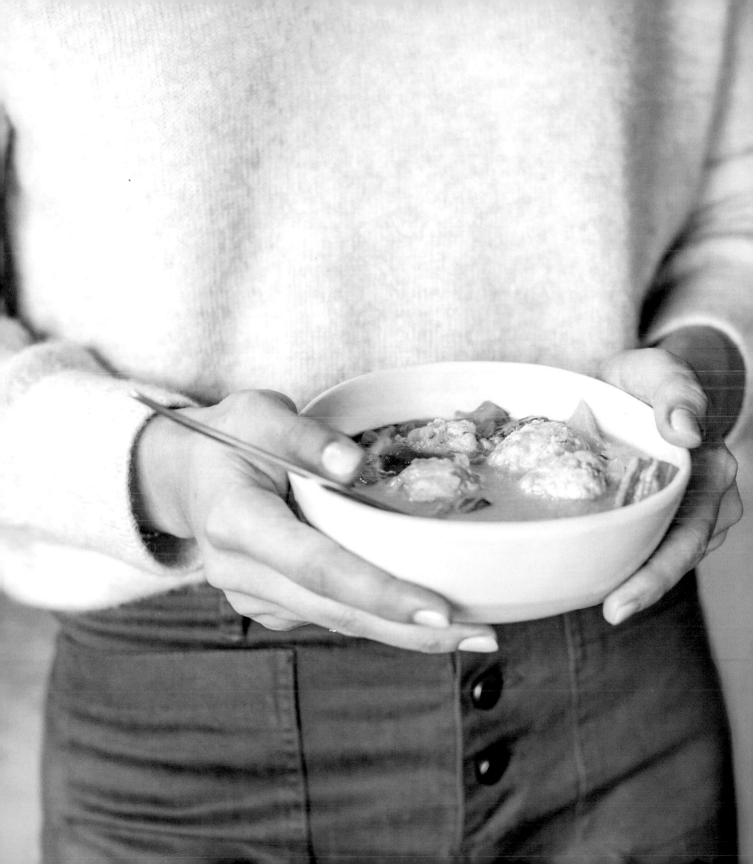

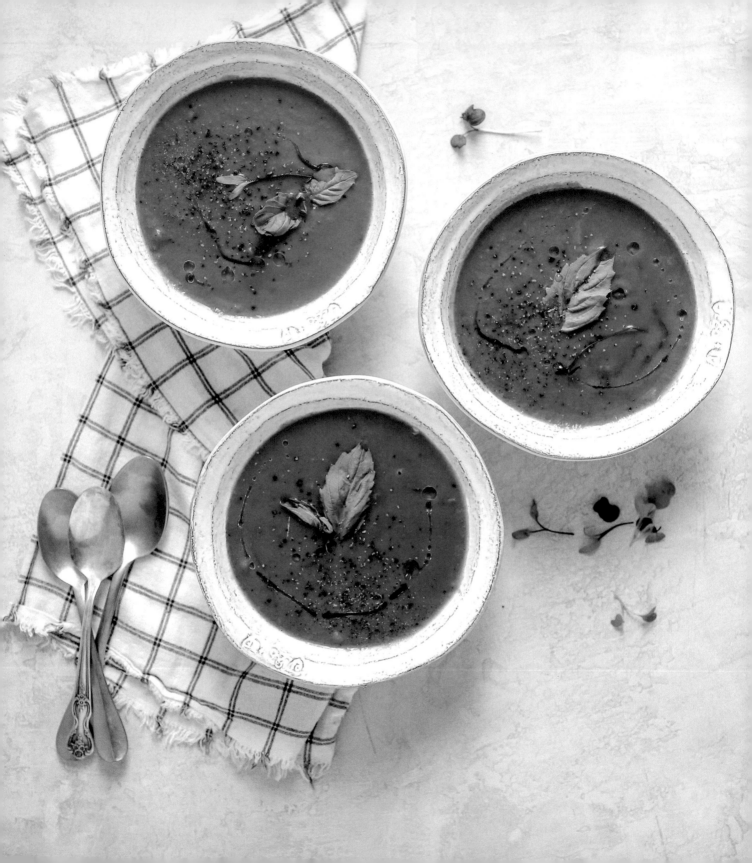

CREAMY TOMATO BASIL SOUP

SERVES 4

➔ GLUTEN-FREE
➔ DAIRY-FREE
➔ PALEO
➔ WHOLE30 IF MODIFIED
➔ GRAIN-FREE

Total time: 25 MINUTES

Growing up, something my dad always made for us on busy weeknights was a bowl of tomato soup with a grilled cheese sandwich. It wasn't anything fancy—the soup was right out of a can—but we absolutely loved it. It's still one of those delicious comfort meals that I crave after a long day, which is why I came up with this version of a creamy tomato soup for my family, which is just as satisfying as Dad's, *almost* as simple, and healthier. Grilled cheese optional!

In a large pot or Dutch oven, heat the olive oil over medium heat. Add the onion, garlic, salt, and pepper and cook until tender, 5 to 7 minutes. Stir in the diced tomatoes, broth, coconut milk, tomato juice, and coconut sugar and bring to a simmer. Cook, uncovered and stirring occasionally, for 15 minutes. Use an immersion blender to puree the soup until smooth, or transfer the soup to a blender in batches and blend until smooth. Taste the soup and season with more salt and pepper, if desired. Stir in the basil. Divide the soup among 4 bowls, drizzle with olive oil, and serve hot.

2 tablespoons extra virgin olive oil, plus more for serving

2 cups diced yellow onion (2 medium)

4 garlic cloves, minced

1 teaspoon kosher salt, or more to taste

½ teaspoon freshly ground black pepper, or more to taste

1 (28-ounce) can diced tomatoes, undrained

1 cup low-sodium chicken or vegetable broth

1 cup unsweetened full-fat coconut milk

1 cup tomato juice

2 tablespoons coconut sugar or balsamic vinegar (see Note)

¼ cup chopped fresh basil leaves

from
MY KITCHEN
to YOURS

The coconut sugar in this recipe helps cut the acidity of the tomatoes. If you want a Whole30 rendition, you can omit the sugar and add 2 tablespoons of aged balsamic vinegar to add a little sweetness to the soup.

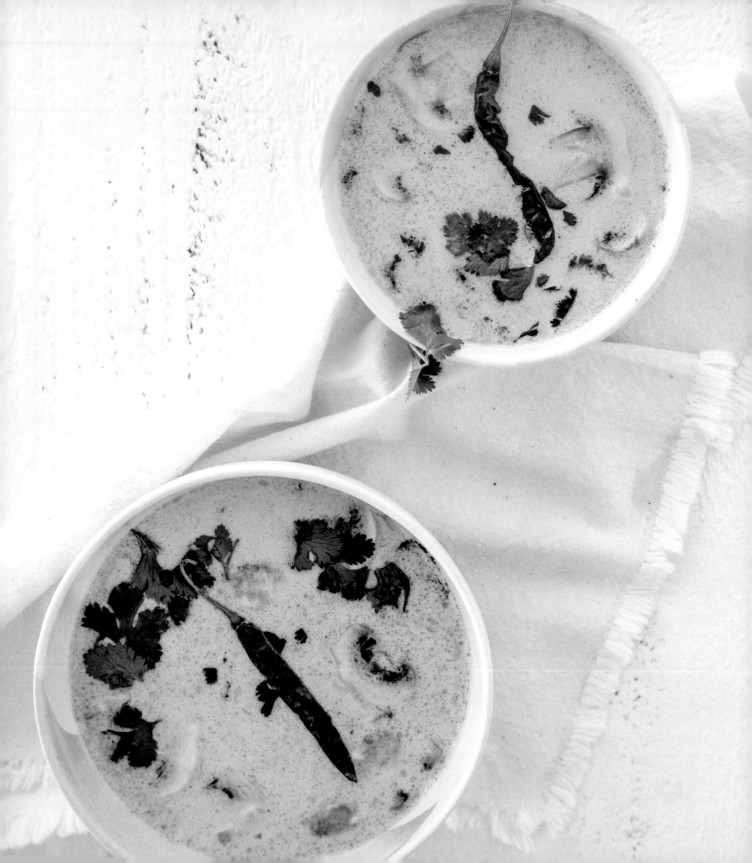

TOM KHA GAI SOUP

SERVES 4

→ GLUTEN-FREE

→ DAIRY-FREE

→ PALEO

→ WHOLE30 IF MODIFIED

→ GRAIN-FREE

Total time: 30 MINUTES

One of my favorite comfort foods of all time is a bowl of Thai coconut soup. This silky, aromatic broth just speaks to me and my soul. I love how simple it is to make, and yet you'll feel like you went out to eat at your favorite Thai restaurant when you take your first bite.

In a large pot or Dutch oven, heat the olive oil over medium heat. Add the shallot and a pinch each of salt and pepper. Cook until the shallots are tender, 2 to 3 minutes. Add the ginger and garlic and cook until fragrant, being careful not to burn, 1 more minute. Add the coconut milk, chicken broth, fish sauce, lime zest, lime juice, coconut sugar, chiles, and coriander. Stir to combine, then add the lemongrass. Bring the soup to a gentle simmer.

Add the sliced chicken and simmer until the chicken is just cooked through, 5 to 6 minutes. Add the mushrooms and simmer for another 3 minutes. Stir in the cilantro and season with salt to taste.

Remove and discard the lemongrass, if desired (I usually just choose to eat around it). Top with the cilantro and serve with lime wedges.

2 tablespoons extra virgin olive oil

½ cup finely diced shallots (2 large)

Kosher salt and freshly ground black pepper

1 (2-inch) piece fresh ginger, grated

2 garlic cloves, minced

2 (13-ounce) cans unsweetened full-fat coconut milk

1 cup low-sodium chicken broth

2 tablespoons fish sauce (I use Red Boat)

Grated zest of ½ lime (1 teaspoon)

3 tablespoons fresh lime juice (about 2 limes)

1 tablespoon coconut palm sugar (omit for Whole30)

2 to 3 bird's eye chiles, very thinly sliced (depending on how spicy you like it)

¼ teaspoon ground coriander

2 stalks of lemongrass (white and light green parts), smashed with the side of a knife and cut into 2-inch pieces

2 pounds boneless, skinless chicken thighs, trimmed and thinly sliced

2 cups thinly sliced white mushrooms

¼ cup fresh cilantro leaves, plus more for serving

1 lime, cut into wedges, for serving

MIMI'S MINESTRA DEL SEDANO

Italian Celery Soup

- 2 tablespoons extra virgin olive oil
- 4 garlic cloves, minced
- 6 large celery stalks (leaves included), cut in ¼-inch slices (4 cups)
- 1 teaspoon kosher salt
- ½ teaspoon freshly ground black pepper
- ¼ teaspoon crushed red pepper flakes (optional)
- 2 (14.5-ounce) cans diced tomatoes, undrained
- 1 (15-ounce) can tomato sauce
- 4 cups low-sodium beef broth or vegetable broth
- 1 cup water
- 2 tablespoons chopped fresh flat-leaf parsley leaves
- 2 tablespoons torn fresh basil leaves
- ½ teaspoon dried oregano
- 2 (15-ounce) cans chickpeas, drained and rinsed
- 1 cup uncooked ditalini or orzo pasta (use gluten-free to keep gluten-free)

This is a recipe that traces back to my great grandmother, if not farther up the family tree. My grandmother, Mimi, made this soup for my mom all the time when she was growing up, and it was in our regular dinner rotation for as long as I can remember. It was one of the first recipes that I called my mom for when I got to college and missed her cooking, and I still have the notes that I jotted down in my little old recipe journal as she recounted it over the phone. Thinking about my ancestors making this dish so long ago just warms my heart, and seeing this little recipe stand the test of time is pure joy. The other great thing about this recipe is that it uses mostly pantry staples and leftovers, making it one of those weeknight meals that you can whip up when you have nothing fresh to make. But don't let that fool you—it's extremely satisfying and simply delicious! I hope you love it as much as my family does.

In a Dutch oven or soup pot, heat the oil over medium heat. Add the garlic, celery, salt, pepper and red pepper flakes (if using) and cook while stirring, until the celery is slightly tender, about 3 minutes. Stir in the diced tomatoes, tomato sauce, broth, water, parsley, basil, and oregano. Increase the heat to medium-high and bring the soup to a boil. Once boiling, reduce the heat to a simmer, cover, and cook, stirring occasionally, until the celery is tender, about 20 minutes.

Add the drained and rinsed chickpeas and the pasta to the soup, stir to combine, cover, and simmer until the pasta is cooked al dente, 8 to 10 minutes. Taste the soup and season with more salt and pepper, if desired.

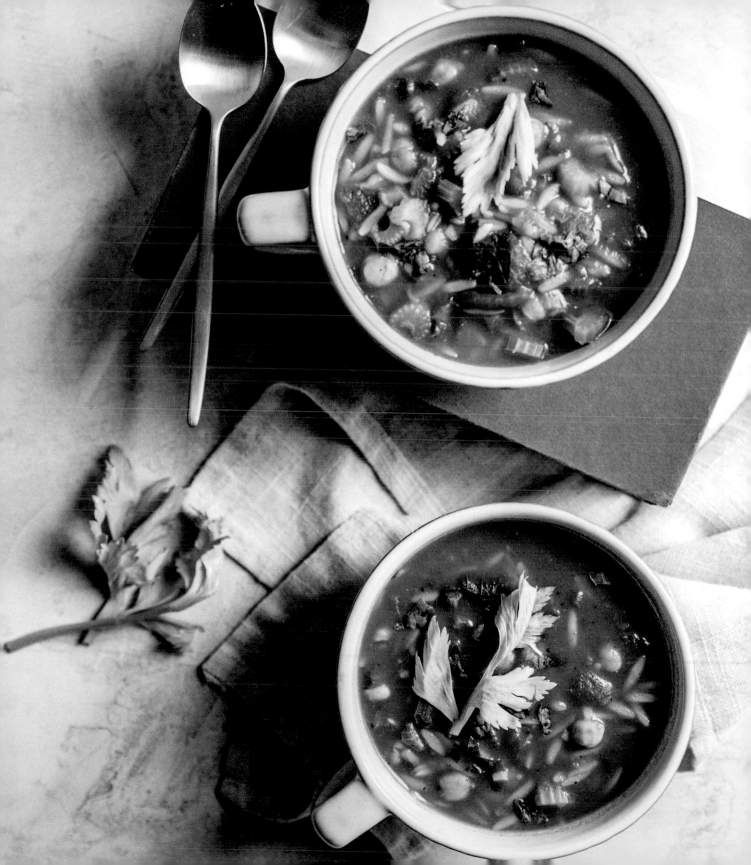

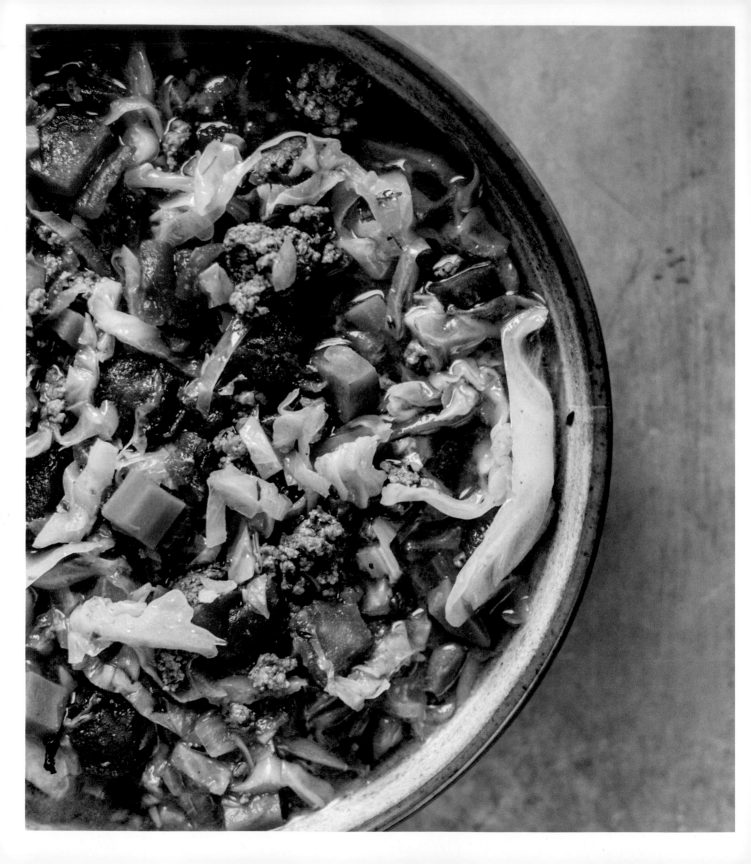

MEXICAN CABBAGE SOUP

SERVES 6

→ GLUTEN-FREE

→ DAIRY-FREE

→ PALEO

→ WHOLE30

→ GRAIN-FREE

Total time: 40 MINUTES

Do you remember when the "cabbage soup diet" was a trend? Basically, people ate cabbage soup for a week to cleanse and detox their bodies? Well, I am not saying I am onboard with that . . . because eating the same thing all week long is certainly not my cup of tea; however, I do like to have a simple cabbage soup for dinner or lunch a few times a week after an indulgent weekend or vacation. It's light, yet satisfying, and it helps boost your metabolism. Plus, this one has an amazing concoction of Mexican-inspired spices that make it taste really wonderful.

In a Dutch oven or large pot, heat the oil over medium-high heat. Add the ground beef, onion, carrot, bell pepper, garlic, salt, and pepper. Cook, breaking up the meat with the back of the spoon, until the beef is no longer pink and the vegetables are tender, about 7 minutes. Drain off the excess fat.

Mix in the broth, cabbage, tomatoes, chili powder, oregano, cayenne pepper, and cumin. Bring to a boil, cover, and reduce to a simmer. Cook until the cabbage is tender, about 20 minutes. Stir in the lime juice, serve, and enjoy!

1 tablespoon extra virgin olive oil

1 pound ground beef, 90 percent lean

½ medium yellow onion, finely diced (1 cup)

1 large carrot, diced (¾ cup)

½ medium green bell pepper, diced (½ cup)

2 garlic cloves, minced

1 teaspoon kosher salt

½ teaspoon freshly ground black pepper

6 cups low-sodium beef broth

½ large head green cabbage, cut in half and thinly sliced (4 cups)

1 (14.5-ounce) can diced fire-roasted tomatoes, undrained

½ teaspoon chili powder

½ teaspoon dried oregano

¼ teaspoon cayenne pepper

¼ teaspoon ground cumin

¼ cup fresh lime juice (about 2 limes)

→ GLUTEN-FREE

→ DAIRY-FREE IF
MODIFIED

→ PALEO IF MODIFIED

→ WHOLE30 IF MODIFIED

→ GRAIN-FREE

Total time: 1 HOUR,
20 MINUTES (8 HOURS USING
THE SLOW COOKER)

TEXAS BRISKET CHILI

3 pounds flat cut brisket, excess
fat trimmed and cut into 1-inch
cubes

1½ teaspoons kosher salt

1 teaspoon freshly ground black
pepper

2 tablespoons extra virgin
olive oil

1 medium yellow onion, diced
(2 cups)

1 medium green bell pepper,
seeded and diced (1½ cups)

4 garlic cloves, minced

2 tablespoons tomato paste

1 teaspoon chili powder

1 teaspoon ground cumin

2 dried bay leaves

1 teaspoon dried oregano

½ teaspoon chipotle chili powder

½ teaspoon smoked paprika

1 (14.5-ounce) can diced
fire-roasted tomatoes

½ cup low-sodium beef broth or
water

¼ cup mild roasted green chiles
(from a jar)

1 tablespoon balsamic vinegar

1 (15-ounce) can pinto beans,
drained and rinsed (omit for
Whole30, paleo)

FOR SERVING (OPTIONAL)
(on following page)

Oh, how I love the taste buds of my fellow Texans: big, bold, and hearty! This Texas-style chili with brisket is no exception. Normally, brisket chili takes all day to cook and uses a combination of dried chiles, but to make life easier (because, *cough*, that's what this book is here for) I used jarred spices and a good-ole Instant Pot to get this rich, beefy stew on the table more quickly and with a lot less work. The end result is everything you've ever dreamed of on a cold day to warm you up. And the best part is that the next day's leftovers are even better! Yee-haw! (Have more time? See below for slow cooker instructions too.)

Season the cubed brisket with the salt and pepper.

Heat the olive oil in an Instant Pot on the sauté function until it shimmers. Working in batches, brown the meat on all sides, about 90 seconds per side. Transfer to a bowl and set aside.

Add the onion, bell pepper, and garlic to the pot and use the sauté function to cook, stirring occasionally, until slightly tender, about 4 minutes. Add the tomato paste, chili powder, cumin, bay leaves, oregano, chipotle chili powder, and paprika and cook while stirring for 1 minute.

Return the browned brisket and all of its juices to the pot along with the fire-roasted tomatoes, broth or water, green chiles, and balsamic vinegar. Stir until well combined, then turn off the heat by hitting the cancel button.

Secure the lid onto the Instant Pot and be sure the vent is sealed. Hit the meat/stew button and set the cook time to

{ continued }

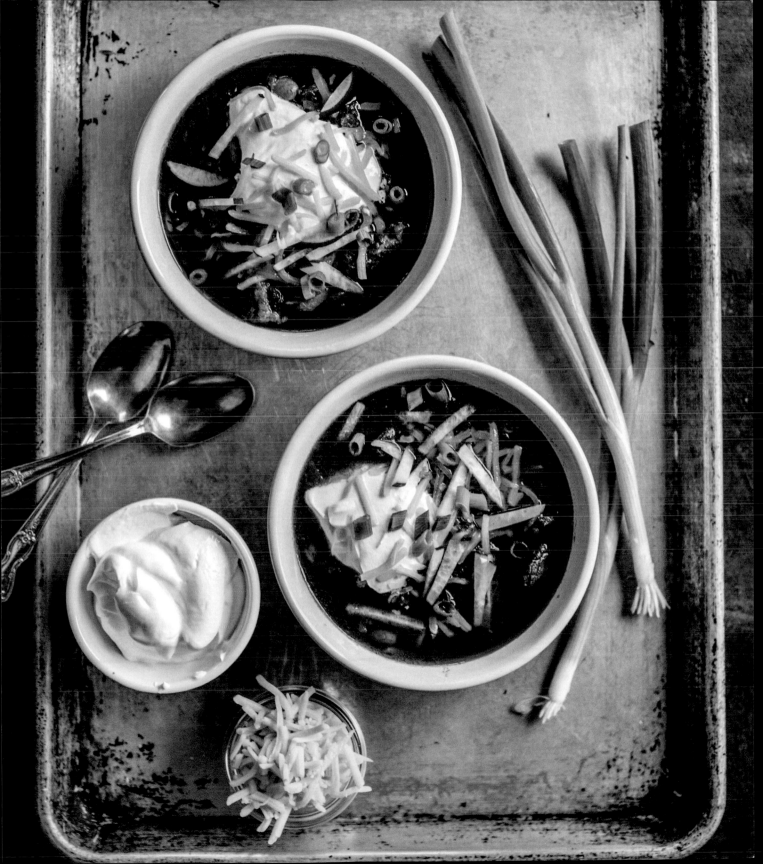

FOR SERVING (OPTIONAL)

2 green onions (green parts only), sliced (½ cup)

2 radishes, cut into matchsticks

½ cup shredded mild cheddar cheese (omit for Whole30, paleo, or dairy-free)

¼ cup sour cream (omit for Whole30, paleo, or dairy-free)

60 minutes on high pressure. When done, carefully release the pressure by turning the valve on top of the Instant Pot. Once the steam has fully released, carefully remove the lid.

Add the drained and rinsed pinto beans (if using) and stir to combine; keep the Instant Pot on warm until heated through, about 5 more minutes. Remove and discard the bay leaves. Serve the chili on its own or topped with green onions, radishes, shredded cheese, and a dollop of sour cream.

SLOW COOKER METHOD

You can also use a slow cooker to make this dish. Just follow the same procedure to sauté the brisket and vegetables in a large skillet over medium-high heat. Transfer the mixture to the slow cooker and add the tomato paste, chili powder, cumin, bay leaves, oregano, chipotle chili powder, paprika, fire-roasted tomatoes, broth or water, green chiles, and balsamic vinegar. Stir to combine, cover, and cook on low for 8 to 10 hours. Stir in the pinto beans and let cook until heated through, about 5 minutes.

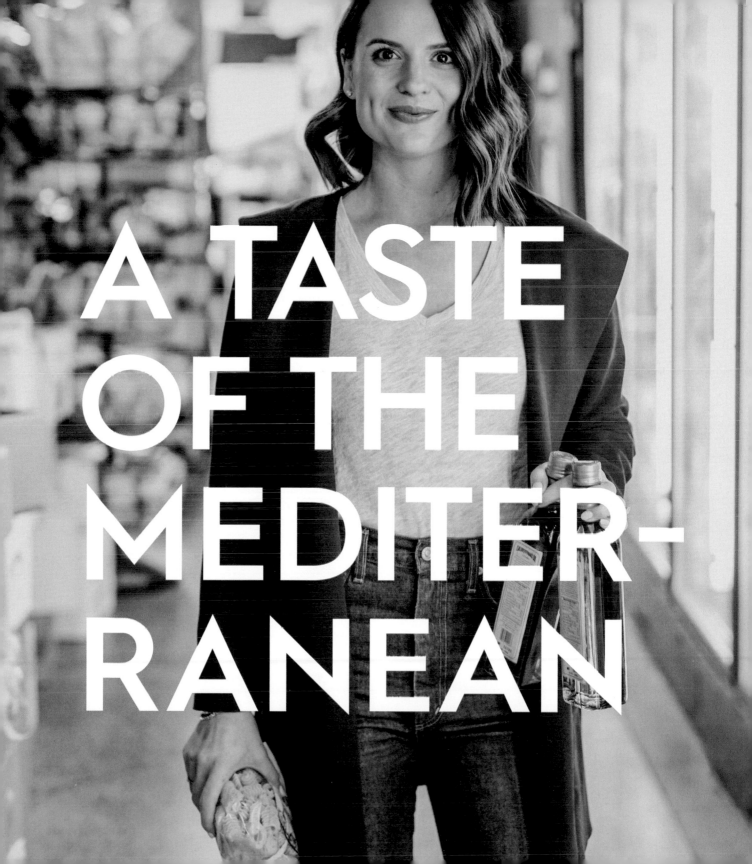

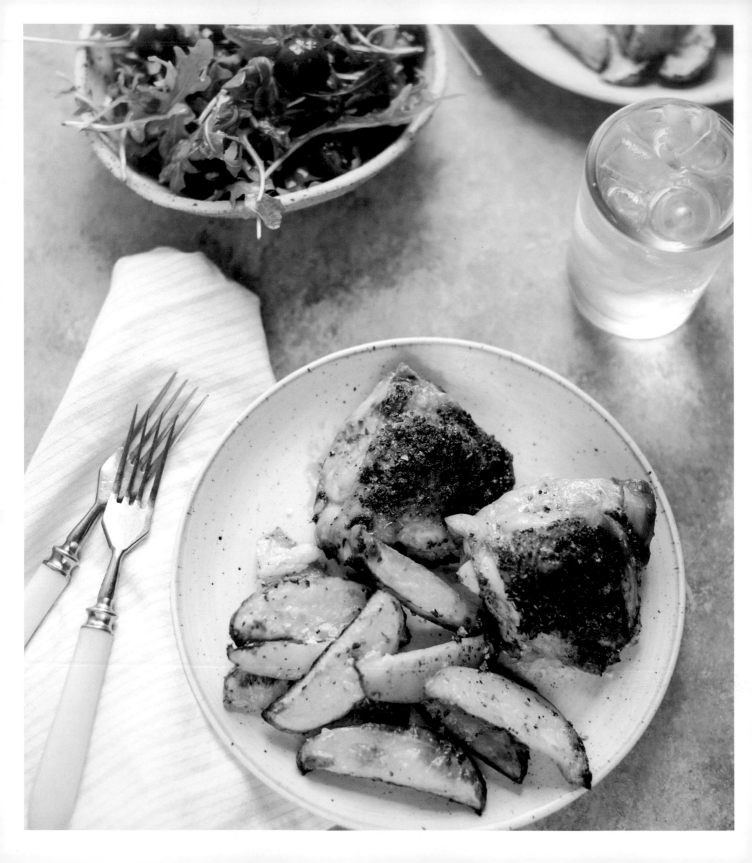

LEMONY GREEK POTATOES *with* CRISPY GREEK CHICKEN THIGHS

SERVES 4

→ GLUTEN-FREE

→ DAIRY-FREE

→ PALEO

→ WHOLE30

→ GRAIN-FREE

Total time: 1 HOUR 15 MINUTES

I absolutely love Greek food because of its bright Mediterranean flavors with lots of fresh citrus and herbs. I especially love Greek potatoes, which are crispy yet tender and tossed with earthy oregano and lemon. Here is my way of getting these amazing potatoes on the table on a busy weeknight, paired with some easy golden chicken thighs. This meal is one that my whole family just adores, so it's a staple on our dinner menu.

MAKE THE POTATOES Preheat the oven to 400°F.

Place the potato wedges in a 9 × 13-inch baking dish. Add the lemon juice, olive oil, broth, salt, oregano, and pepper and mix until evenly combined. Spread the potatoes into a single even layer and bake, gently tossing every 20 minutes, until tender and golden brown, about 1 hour total.

MAKE THE CHICKEN Line a large baking sheet with parchment paper. While the potatoes bake, arrange the chicken thighs on the baking sheet in a single even layer. Make sure they are not touching. Pat dry the tops of the chicken thighs, then drizzle each thigh with olive oil to coat.

In a small bowl, mix together the paprika, salt, oregano, and pepper until well combined, then sprinkle evenly over the chicken.

Bake the chicken until it is cooked through and the skin is crispy and golden brown, 35 to 45 minutes, depending on the size. Let the chicken cool for 10 minutes before serving.

FOR THE GREEK POTATOES

- 1½ pounds Yukon gold potatoes (4 medium potatoes), halved lengthwise and sliced into ¼-inch wedges
- ⅓ cup fresh lemon juice (2 lemons)
- ¼ cup extra virgin olive oil
- ¼ cup low-sodium chicken broth
- 1½ teaspoons kosher salt
- 1 teaspoon dried oregano
- ½ teaspoon freshly ground black pepper

FOR THE CHICKEN

- 2 pounds bone-in, skin-on chicken thighs
- 2 tablespoons extra virgin olive oil
- 1 teaspoon smoked paprika
- 1 teaspoon kosher salt
- ½ teaspoon dried oregano
- ½ teaspoon freshly ground black pepper

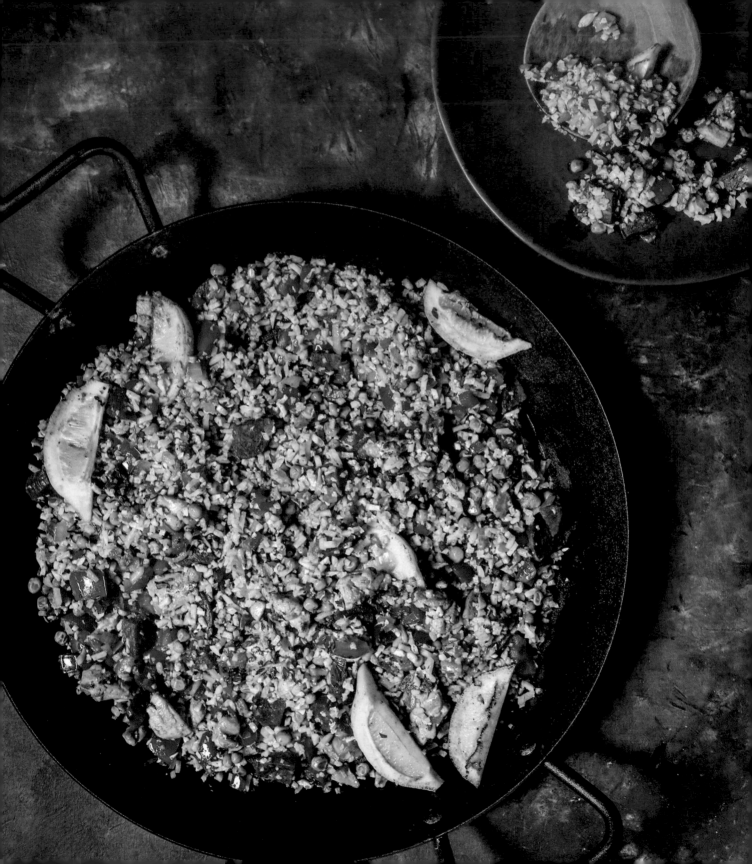

CHORIZO *and* CHICKEN PAELLA

SERVES 4
→ GLUTEN-FREE
→ DAIRY-FREE
→ PALEO IF MODIFIED
→ WHOLE30 IF MODIFIED
→ GRAIN-FREE
Total time: 40 MINUTES

My junior year of college I studied abroad in Seville, Spain. It was one of the most transformative experiences of my life and one I will always cherish. During that time I ate a lot of paella, a traditional saffron-spiced rice dish that's loaded with chorizo, chicken, and shrimp. "When in Rome," right?! This recipe is a decidedly *untraditional* take on paella because it calls for using cauliflower rice instead of the usual Bomba or short-grain rice, but the flavor is still layered and delicious. I understand if you're skeptical—the first time I made this, my husband said, "By the sound of it, I can already tell you that I'm not going to like it." Two bowls later, he confessed that it was "really freaking good." And that it is! It's all the flavors of paella in a delicious, low-carb weeknight meal.

In a large skillet or paella pan, heat the oil over medium-high heat. Add the cubed chicken, 1 teaspoon of salt, and the black pepper. Cook the chicken, tossing occasionally, until cooked through and golden brown around the edges, about 7 minutes. Use a slotted spoon to transfer the cooked chicken to a plate. Set aside.

Add the chorizo, onion, bell pepper, and garlic to the same skillet and cook, stirring, until the onion and peppers have softened, 3 to 4 minutes. Add the paprika and cook, stirring, for 1 more minute. Add the wine and saffron, and cook, stirring occasionally, until the liquid is reduced by half, about 2 minutes.

Reduce the heat to medium and return chicken back to the skillet, along with the cauliflower rice and peas. Stir to combine and cook, stirring until the cauliflower is just heated through, 4 to 6 minutes. Add the remaining ½ teaspoon salt, plus more to taste, if desired. Stir in the tomato and parsley. Remove the pan from the heat and serve with the lemon wedges.

- 2 tablespoons extra virgin olive oil
- 4 boneless, skinless chicken thighs, trimmed and cut into ½-inch cubes
- 1½ teaspoons kosher salt
- ½ teaspoon freshly ground black pepper
- 6 ounces cured Spanish-style chorizo sausage, casing removed, quartered lengthwise, and sliced
- 1 cup finely diced yellow onion (1 medium)
- ¾ cup finely diced red bell pepper (1 small)
- 2 garlic cloves, finely chopped
- 1 teaspoon smoked paprika
- ½ cup dry white wine (substitute low-sodium chicken broth for Whole30, paleo)
- ½ teaspoon saffron threads (15 to 20 threads)
- 4 cups riced cauliflower, preferably fresh not frozen
- ½ cup frozen peas (omit for Whole30)
- 1 Roma tomato, seeded and diced small
- 2 tablespoons chopped fresh flat-leaf parsley leaves
- 1 lemon, cut into wedges, for serving

SERVES 4

→ GLUTEN-FREE

→ DAIRY-FREE

→ PALEO

→ WHOLE30

→ GRAIN-FREE

Total time: 45 MINUTES

SHEET PAN SAUSAGE *with* SQUASH *and* ROASTED GRAPES

3 cups delicata or acorn squash (or 1 large squash) cut in half lengthwise, seeds removed and cut into ¼-inch slices

2 cups thinly sliced yellow onion (2 medium)

2 cups red grapes

3 tablespoons extra virgin olive oil

1 teaspoon herbes de Provence

1 teaspoon kosher salt

½ teaspoon freshly ground black pepper

1½ pounds sweet, mild, or hot Italian pork sausage

1 lemon, cut into wedges, for serving

Have you ever tried roasted grapes? I absolutely love them and grapes are always something I have in my fridge since they are one of my kids' favorite snacks. When roasted, they are delectable, sweet, and juicy. Here in this simple weeknight sheet pan dish I combine these delicious roasted grapes with Italian sausages, delicata squash, and herbes de Provence for a simple, sweet, and savory dish that you'll just love!

Preheat the oven to 400°F and line a large baking sheet with parchment paper.

Place the delicata squash, onion, and grapes on the prepared baking sheet. Drizzle with the olive oil and sprinkle with the herbes de Provence, salt, and black pepper. Toss until the vegetables and grapes are evenly coated.

Nestle the sausages in with the vegetable mixture, rubbing the sausages with the olive oil in the sheet pan so they are lightly coated with oil. Arrange the vegetables around the sausages so they are spread in one even layer.

Place in the preheated oven and bake in oven until the sausages are cooked through and the squash is tender, about 35 minutes, flipping sausages halfway through the cooking process.

Remove from the oven and serve with lemon wedges.

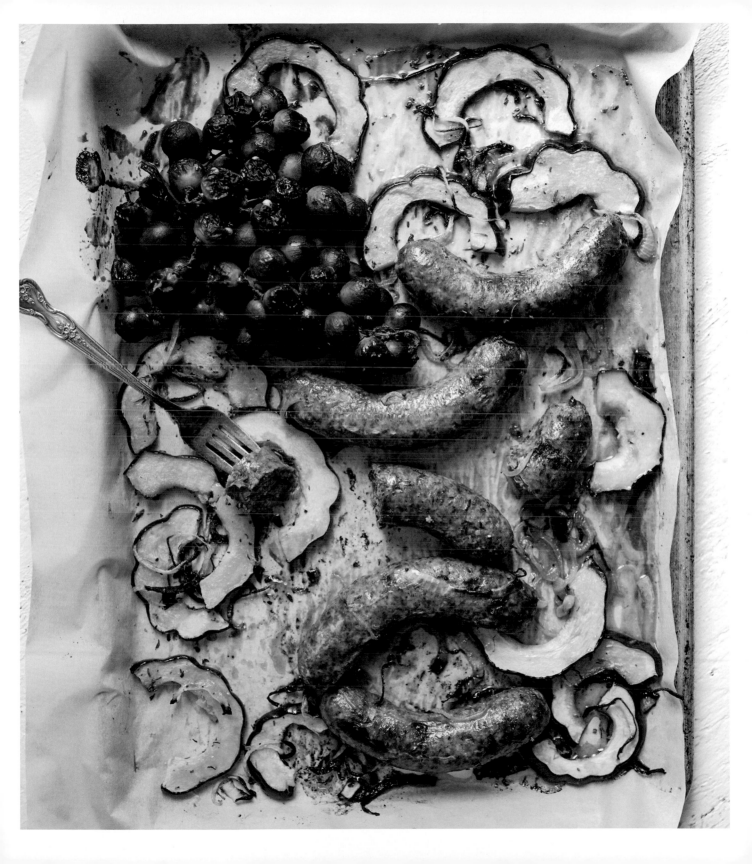

MUSSELS *with* SAFFRON *and* FENNEL BROTH

2 tablespoons extra virgin olive oil

2 medium fennel bulbs, quartered and thinly sliced crosswise (1 cup)

½ cup finely diced yellow onion (½ medium)

1 teaspoon kosher salt

½ teaspoon freshly ground black pepper

2 garlic cloves, minced

1½ cups dry white wine (see Note)

½ teaspoon saffron threads (15 to 20 threads)

¼ teaspoon crushed red pepper flakes (optional)

¾ cup low-sodium chicken broth

2 pounds mussels, scrubbed and debearded

2 tablespoons finely chopped fresh flat-leaf parsley leaves

Crusty bread, rice, Prepared Cauliflower Rice (page 282), or zucchini noodles, for serving

Mussels in a saffron broth might sound like a strictly-for-restaurants dish, but believe me when I tell you that you easily make this at home! Although serving this with crusty bread to soak up all of the delicious broth is a pretty magical pairing, it's not necessary if you are trying to avoid gluten or grains. This dish is great served over rice, cauliflower rice, or zucchini noodles.

In a large saucepan, heat the olive oil over medium heat. Add the fennel, onion, salt, and pepper. Cook until the fennel and onion are tender, 3 to 4 minutes. Add the garlic and gently cook, stirring, until fragrant, about 1 more minute.

Increase the heat to medium-high and add the wine, saffron, and red pepper flakes (if using). Cook until the wine has reduced by half, 2 to 3 minutes. Pour in the broth and bring to a simmer. Carefully add the mussels and gently toss to coat in the sauce. Cover and cook, shaking the pan occasionally to evenly cook the mussels, until the mussels begin to open, about 5 minutes.

Use a slotted spoon to transfer the mussels into a large serving bowl, discarding any of the mussels that have not opened. Pour the broth over the mussels. Garnish with parsley and serve with bread, rice, cauliflower rice, or zucchini noodles.

from
MY KITCHEN
to YOURS

If you're Whole30 or paleo, substitute an additional 1½ cups low-sodium chicken broth plus the juice of 1 lemon for the white wine.

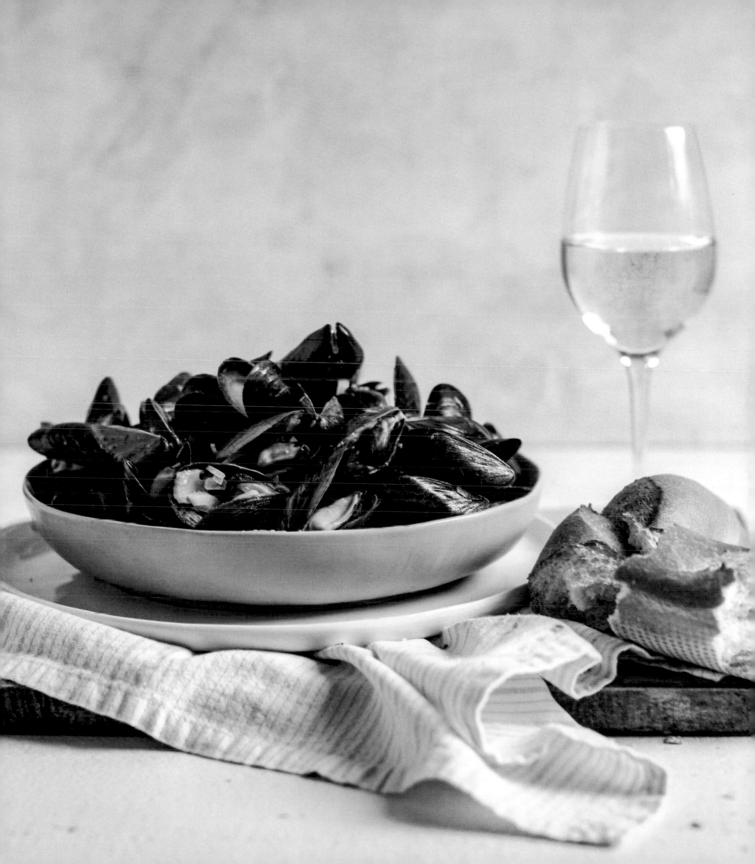

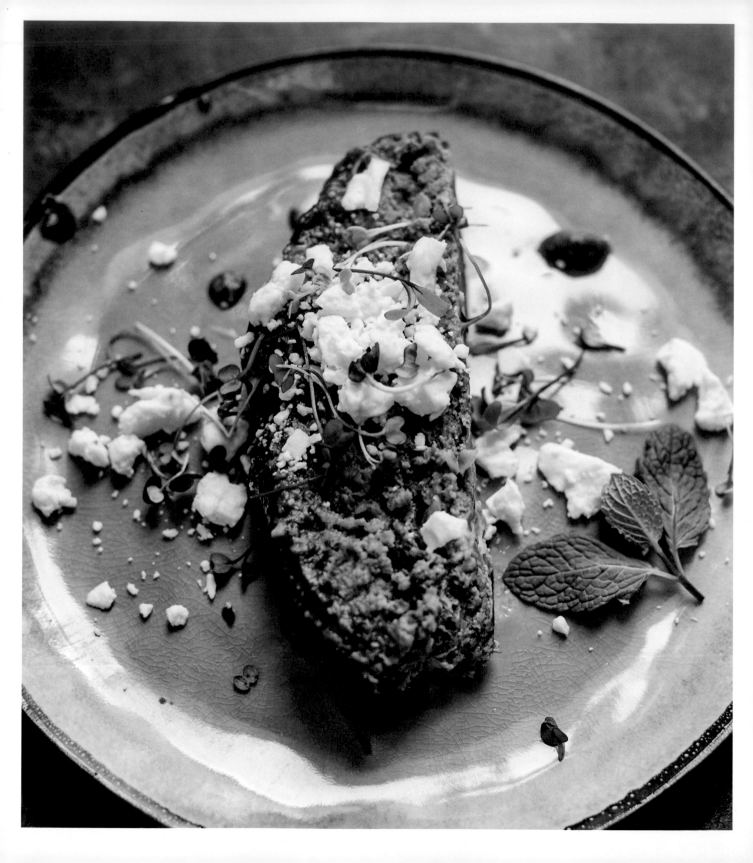

GREEK-STYLE MEATLOAF

SERVES 6

→ GLUTEN-FREE

→ DAIRY-FREE IF MODIFIED

→ PALEO IF MODIFIED

→ WHOLE30 IF MODIFIED

→ GRAIN-FREE

Total time: 1 HOUR, 30 MINUTES

You've probably noticed by now that my husband is my biggest fan—I mention him a lot! He is what I like to call my "Gordon Ramsay" because he is brutally honest about everything that I make, which is great because it's exactly the feedback I need. And when Clayton loves a dish, I *know* it's a hit! When he took a bite of this meatloaf, his exact words were, "This is the best meatloaf I've ever tasted." It is some dang good meatloaf with all of the fabulous Greek-inspired ingredients we all love, like lamb, oregano, mint, and feta.

MAKE THE MEATLOAF Preheat the oven to 350°F. Line a large sheet pan with parchment paper and set aside.

Melt the ghee in a large skillet over medium heat. Add the onions and 1 teaspoon of the oregano and cook, stirring, until the onion is tender, about 7 minutes. Remove from the heat and stir in the tomato paste and balsamic vinegar. Set aside to cool.

In a large bowl, combine the ground beef, ground lamb, eggs, almond flour, mint, parsley, the remaining 1 teaspoon oregano, salt, and pepper. Fold in the cooled onion mixture and the feta cheese (if using) and use a fork to lightly mix—don't mash the meat, or it will be dense. Form the mixture into an oval-shaped loaf on the prepared sheet pan. It should be about 10 inches long and 2 inches thick.

MAKE THE SAUCE In a small bowl, whisk together the tomato sauce, mustard, garlic, tomato paste, balsamic vinegar, salt, and cayenne pepper. Spread the sauce all over the top and sides of the meatloaf.

Bake the meatloaf for 1 hour, or until a meat thermometer inserted into the center of the meatloaf registers 155°F. Let rest for 10 minutes before cutting into thick slices and serving.

FOR THE MEATLOAF

- 2 tablespoons ghee
- 2 cups finely diced yellow onion (1 large)
- 2 teaspoons dried oregano
- 1 tablespoon tomato paste
- 1 tablespoon balsamic vinegar
- 1 pound ground beef, 85 percent lean
- 1 pound ground lamb
- 2 large eggs, beaten
- ½ cup almond flour
- 2 tablespoons fresh mint leaves, finely chopped
- 2 tablespoons finely chopped fresh flat-leaf parsley leaves
- 1 teaspoon kosher salt
- ½ teaspoon freshly ground black pepper
- ½ cup crumbled feta cheese (omit for Whole30, paleo, dairy-free)

FOR THE SAUCE

- ½ cup tomato sauce
- 2 tablespoons stone ground mustard
- 2 garlic cloves, minced
- 1 tablespoon tomato paste
- 1 tablespoon balsamic vinegar
- ½ teaspoon kosher salt
- ⅛ teaspoon cayenne pepper

SERVES 4

→ GLUTEN-FREE

→ GRAIN-FREE

Total time: 40 MINUTES

SUMAC-ROASTED SALMON *with* MINT-CORIANDER YOGURT SAUCE

FOR THE SUMAC-ROASTED SALMON

- 1 (2-pound) king salmon fillet, bones removed
- 2 tablespoons extra virgin olive oil
- 1 teaspoon ground sumac
- ½ teaspoon kosher salt
- ½ teaspoon freshly ground black pepper

FOR THE MINT-CORIANDER YOGURT SAUCE

- ½ cup plain nonfat Greek yogurt
- 2 garlic cloves, minced
- 2 tablespoons finely chopped fresh mint leaves
- 2 tablespoons extra virgin olive oil
- 1 tablespoon fresh lemon juice (½ lemon)
- ¼ teaspoon ground coriander
- ¼ teaspoon kosher salt
- ⅛ teaspoon freshly ground black pepper

- 1 lemon, cut into wedges, for serving

If you've never cooked with sumac—or never heard of it— it's time to get out and find you some! Sumac is a dried red spice traditionally used in Middle Eastern cooking. Made by crushing the dried fruits of the sumac bush, ground sumac has a bright, tart flavor that helps highlight other flavors in a dish while adding an unexpected pop of complexity and freshness (especially to simple ingredients, like the salmon in this dish). Your local supermarket may not carry it, but it's worth seeking out, whether it be at your local specialty grocer or online.

MAKE THE SALMON Preheat the oven to 375°F. Line a large baking sheet with parchment paper and set aside.

Lay the salmon skin-side down on the prepared baking sheet. Brush with the oil to evenly coat the top, then season the top evenly with the sumac, salt, and pepper. Roast until the salmon is flaky and cooked through, about 30 minutes.

MAKE THE YOGURT SAUCE While the salmon cooks, in a medium bowl combine the yogurt, garlic, mint, olive oil, lemon juice, coriander, salt, and pepper. Stir until well combined and refrigerate until ready to serve.

Divide the salmon between four plates, top with your desired amount of yogurt sauce, and serve with a wedge of lemon.

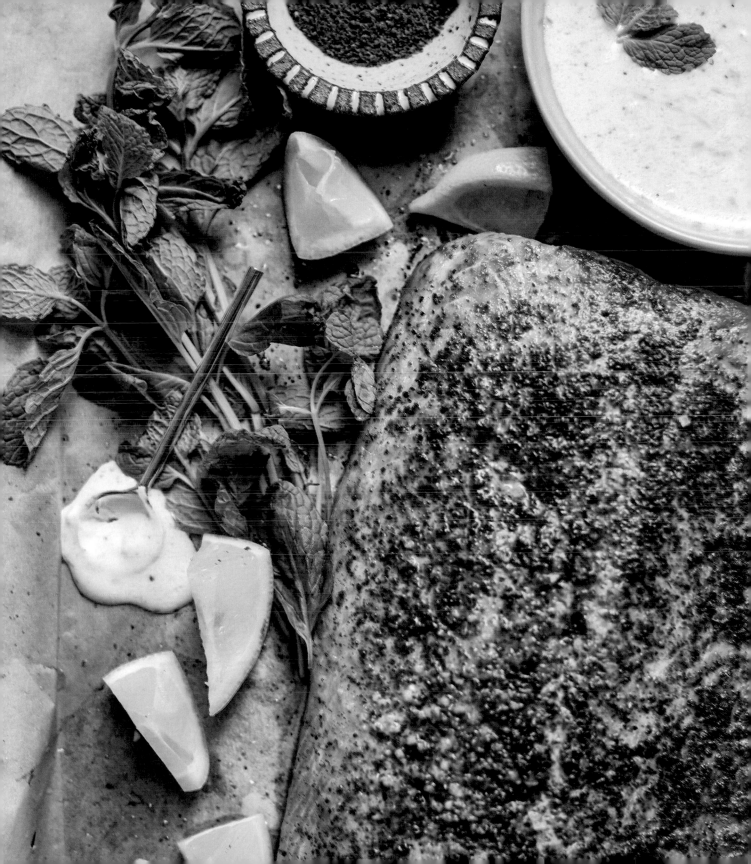

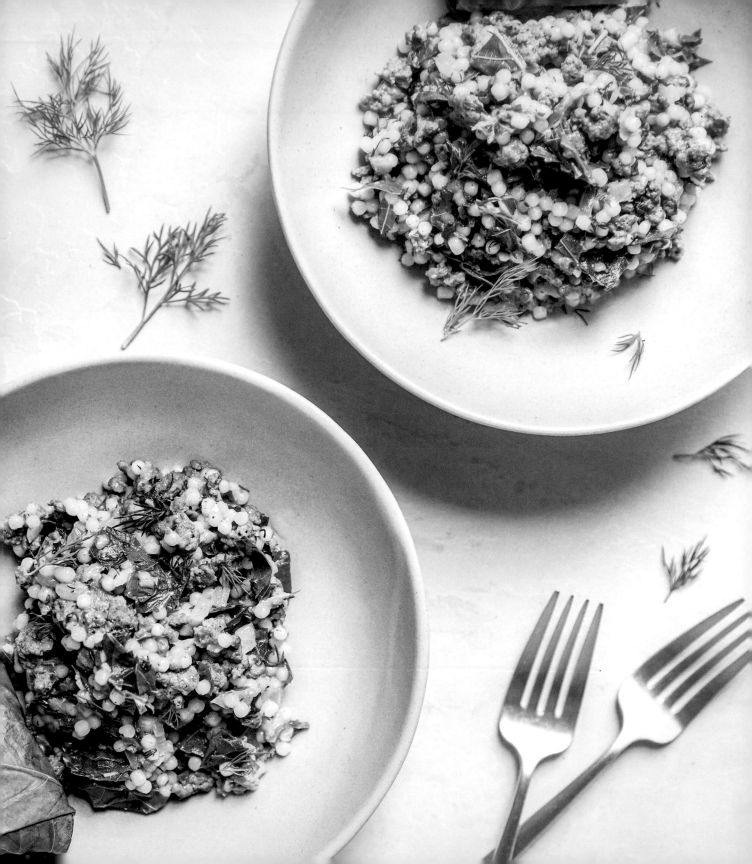

ONE-POT UNSTUFFED GRAPE LEAVES

SERVES 4

→ DAIRY-FREE

Total time: 30 MINUTES

Dolmas, or stuffed grape leaves, are one of my most admired Greek delicacies. I adore the delicious dill and lemon flavors packed into each grape leaf. I could just eat them like candy! Although delicious, grape leaf rolling at home on a busy weeknight is a pretty daunting and time-consuming task, which is why I've packed all the flavors into this one-pot wonder! If you love dolmas and vibrant Greek flavors, you are going to absolutely love this dish.

Heat the olive oil in a skillet over medium-high heat. When the oil is shimmering, add the onion and garlic and cook, stirring, until tender, 3 to 4 minutes. Add the lamb, oregano, crushed red pepper flakes, salt, and pepper and cook, breaking up the meat with the back of a spoon, until cooked through (or no longer pink), 5 to 7 minutes. Drain off excess fat and return the browned beef to the skillet on over medium-high heat.

Add the couscous, grape leaves, chicken broth, and lemon juice and stir to combine. Bring to a boil and reduce until simmering. Cook, stirring often, until the liquid is absorbed and couscous is tender, 10 to 12 minutes.

Once couscous is cooked and tender, add the dill, mint, and parsley and stir to combine. Taste and add more salt and pepper, if desired.

Serve with a wedge of lemon and enjoy!

- 2 tablespoons extra virgin olive oil
- 1 cup finely diced yellow onion (½ medium)
- 4 cloves garlic, minced
- 1 pound ground lamb (or 90 percent lean ground beef)
- ½ teaspoon dried oregano
- ¼ teaspoon crushed red pepper flakes
- 1 teaspoon kosher salt
- ½ teaspoon freshly ground black pepper
- 1 cup uncooked Israeli couscous
- 1 (6-ounce) jar grape leaves, drained, rinsed and loosely chopped (about 1 cup)
- 2 cups low sodium chicken broth
- ¼ cup fresh lemon juice (about 2 lemons)
- 2 tablespoons finely chopped fresh dill
- 2 tablespoons finely chopped fresh mint leaves
- 2 tablespoons finely chopped fresh flat-leaf parsley leaves
- 1 lemon, cut into wedges, for serving

MEDITERRANEAN FISH *en* PAPILLÔTE

5 ounces haricots verts

1 clove garlic, very thinly sliced

2 fillets petrale sole (or other white flaky fish like halibut, cod, or tilapia)

2 tablespoons extra virgin olive oil

½ teaspoon kosher salt

¼ teaspoon freshly ground black pepper

½ lemon, sliced into ¼-inch rounds

½ cup cherry tomatoes, halved

¼ cup Kalamata olives, halved

1 tablespoon fresh oregano leaves

Fish in Parchment Paper

Fish cooked *en papillôte,* or in parchment paper, is an easy, healthy, and flavorful way to cook fish. In this recipe, lemon, herbs, veggies, and fish are tucked away in a folded parchment pouch to create a light and flavorful dinner. Not only is it easy to cook, but it's equally easy to clean up—one reason why it's probably one of my favorite methods to cook fish, and absolutely perfect for weeknights.

Preheat the oven to 400°F and lay out two 9 × 11-inch pieces of parchment paper on a flat surface.

Evenly divide the haricots verts and sliced garlic among the two pieces of parchment paper, placing the ingredients in the center of the parchment. Place the sole on top of the haricots verts and drizzle each fillet with 1 tablespoon olive oil. Season with salt and pepper and evenly distribute the lemon, cherry tomatoes, olives, and oregano over the top of the sole fillets.

Fold down the short ends of the parchment paper over the fish, making a rectangle. Then, grab the open ends and roll towards the fish, so that no liquids can escape and creating an enclosed package.

Place the parcels in a 9 x 13-inch baking dish and place in oven. Bake until the fish is cooked through and flakes easily, about 15 minutes.

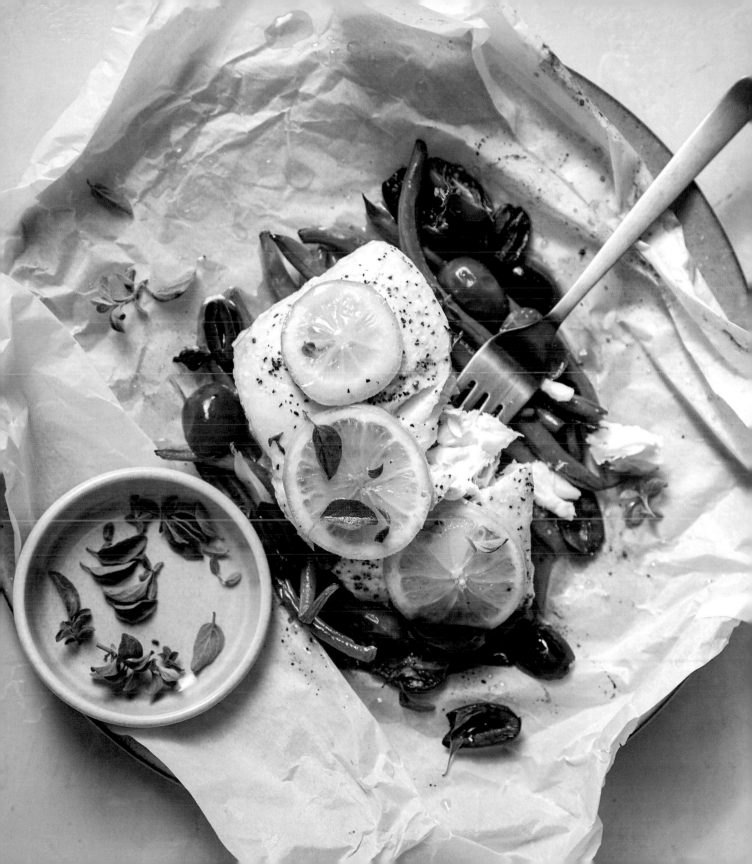

SERVES 4

→ GLUTEN-FREE

→ DAIRY-FREE

→ PALEO IF MODIFIED

→ WHOLE30 IF MODIFIED

→ GRAIN-FREE

Total time: 40 MINUTES

SOLOMILLO AL WHISKY

Seville-Style Pork with Garlic and Whiskey

1 pound pork tenderloin

1½ teaspoon kosher salt

½ teaspoons freshly ground black pepper

2 tablespoons arrowroot starch

3 tablespoons extra virgin olive oil

8 garlic cloves, peeled then smashed

⅓ cup cognac or whiskey (substitute chicken broth for Whole30, paleo)

1 pound yellow potatoes, peeled and cut into ½-inch cubes

2½ cups low-sodium chicken broth

1 tablespoon apple cider vinegar

½ teaspoon paprika

2 tablespoons fresh lemon juice (1 lemon)

1 teaspoon chopped fresh flat-leaf parsley leaves, for garnish

I will never forget my first week studying abroad in Seville, Spain, scanning a menu and thinking: *What the heck does this say and what should I order?* Being the foodie that I am, I began asking locals about their favorite traditional dishes. I knew I had to try *Solomillo al Whisky* after one of my professors passionately described the dish and its flavors to me. After class, I headed to the restaurant that he recommended and placed an order . . . and wow! He was right. This famous Seville dish is absolutely delicious! Pork and potatoes cooked in a garlicky whiskey sauce make a fantastic flavor combination and a great, comforting weeknight meal. Although nothing will ever beat enjoying this dish on the streets of Seville, I've adapted it for my home kitchen to cue all of the nostalgic feelings of my time spent there.

Slice the pork tenderloin into ½-inch medallions.

Lay the medallions on a cutting board and cover with a sheet of parchment paper. Using a meat mallet or the bottom of a skillet, gently pound until the medallions are ¼ inch thin. Season both sides of the medallions with 1 teaspoon of the salt and the pepper.

Place the arrowroot on a plate. Place each medallion in the flour and dredge until both sides are coated in the arrowroot. Shake off excess and set aside. Continue until all of the medallions are dredged.

{ continued }

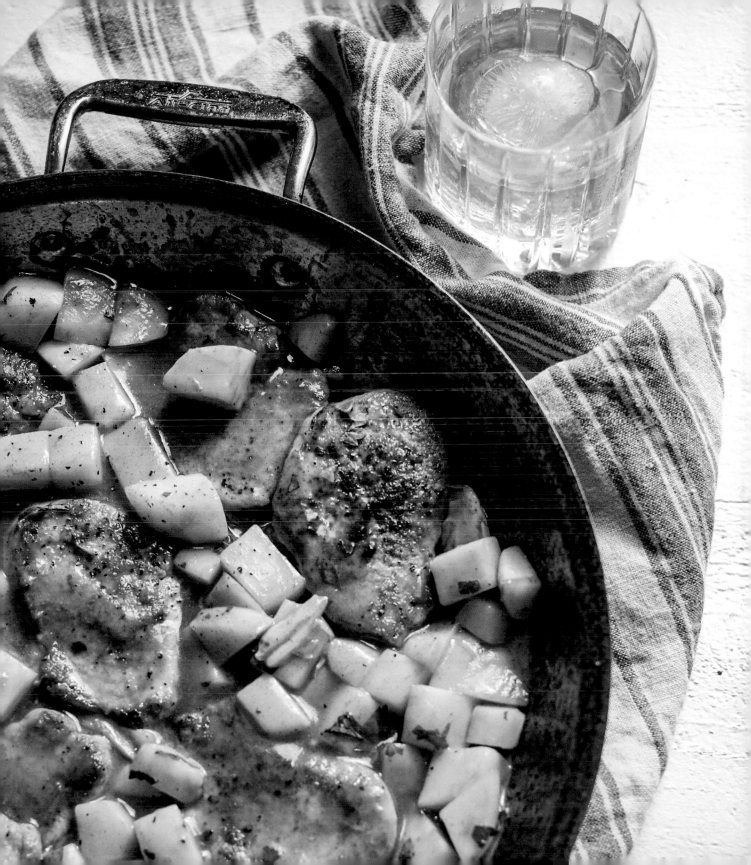

Heat a large skillet with tall sides over medium-high heat with 2 tablespoons olive oil. When hot, sear both sides of the medallions until golden brown, 2 to 3 minutes per side. Do not overcrowd the pan to allow the medallions to brown nicely; you may need to do this in two batches depending on the size of your skillet. As they are browned, set aside the medallions on a plate.

Reduce the heat to medium and add the remaining 1 tablespoon olive oil and the garlic. Cook, stirring, until fragrant, being careful not to burn the garlic, about 1 minute. Add the whiskey to the skillet and use a wooden spoon to scrape up all the brown bits. Cook until the whiskey has nearly completely evaporated, about 1 minute. Add the potatoes and the remaining ½ teaspoon salt and toss to coat in the little bit of liquid in the skillet.

Pour in 2 cups of the broth and the apple cider vinegar and stir to combine. Nestle the medallions back into the skillet and bring to a boil. Once boiling, reduce the heat to a light simmer, cover, and cook, stirring occasionally, until the sauce has thickened, about 10 minutes. Once the sauce is thick, add the remaining ½ cup broth, the paprika, and the lemon juice and stir to combine. Cover and continue to cook, gently simmering, until the potatoes are fork tender, about 10 more minutes.

Garnish with freshly chopped parsley and add more salt and pepper to taste, if desired.

OVEN-BAKED CHICKEN KOFTA WRAPS

SERVES 6

→ GLUTEN-FREE

→ DAIRY-FREE

→ PALEO

→ WHOLE30

→ GRAIN-FREE

Total time: 60 MINUTES

Kofta is a Middle Eastern dish made from ground lamb or beef mixed with warm spices like paprika, cumin, allspice, and cinnamon. The mixture is shaped into balls or patties, grilled, and served with pita, salads, dips, and sauces. To get them on skewers and to get them to hold together on a grill can be a little tricky, so I've come up with a foolproof oven-baked version. You may have to get your hands a little dirty for this dish, but boy-oh-boy is it worth it! These little chicken kofta patties are easy to make if you follow these simple steps—and talk about delicious flavors! I love serving mine in lettuce cups filled with cucumbers, tomatoes, and a delicious lemon-garlic aioli.

MAKE THE CHICKEN KOFTA Preheat the oven to 375°F. Line 2 large baking sheets with parchment paper and set aside.

In a food processor or blender, combine the onion, parsley, and garlic. Process until the onion and parsley are finely minced, almost to a pulp. Transfer to a sieve or fine mesh strainer. Press down on the mixture with the back of a spoon, draining off any excess liquid.

In a large bowl, combine the ground chicken breast, ground chicken thigh, egg, salt, paprika, cumin, allspice, turmeric, black pepper, cayenne pepper, and cinnamon. Add the onion-parsley pulp to the bowl and begin kneading the mixture with your hands. After a few minutes, it will have a sticky, paste-like consistency.

Use a 1.25 ounce (2.5 tablespoons/#30) scoop to scoop the mixture onto the prepared baking sheets about 1½ inches apart.

{ continued }

FOR THE CHICKEN KOFTA

- 1 small yellow onion, cut into eight wedges
- 2 cups loosely packed fresh curly parsley
- 3 garlic cloves
- 1 pound ground chicken breast
- 1 pound ground chicken thigh
- 1 large egg
- 1½ teaspoons kosher salt
- ½ teaspoon paprika
- ½ teaspoon ground cumin
- ½ teaspoon allspice
- ½ teaspoon ground turmeric
- ½ teaspoon freshly ground black pepper
- ¼ teaspoon cayenne pepper
- ¼ teaspoon ground cinnamon

FOR THE LEMON-GARLIC AIOLI

- ½ cup homemade mayo (page 281)
- Grated zest of ½ lemon (1 teaspoon)
- 2 tablespoons fresh lemon juice (1 lemon)
- 2 garlic cloves, minced
- ¼ teaspoon kosher salt

TO ASSEMBLE
(on following page)

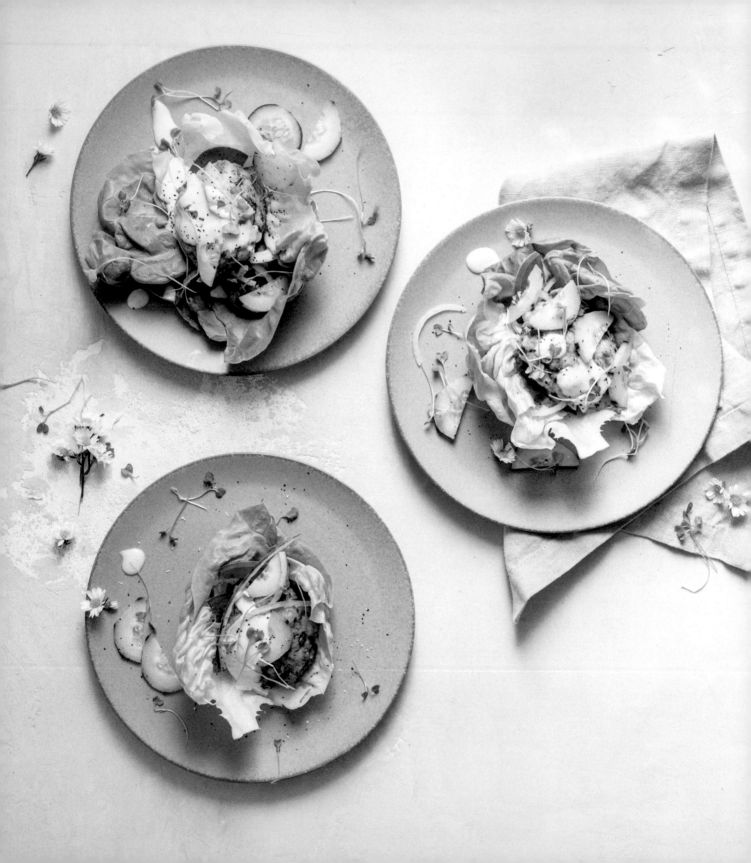

TO ASSEMBLE

1 head butter lettuce

1 hothouse cucumber, peeled, halved lengthwise, and cut into thin slices

2 ripe tomatoes, halved and thinly sliced

½ red onion, thinly sliced (1 cup)

With damp hands, flatten the tops of the koftas and round out the sides, forming them into uniform patties. (Damp hands help make working with the sticky, paste-like meat easier.)

Bake for 20 to 25 minutes, until the kofta patties are cooked through, or no longer pink when cut through the center, and golden brown. Let the koftas cool slightly before assembling.

MAKE THE LEMON-GARLIC AIOLI In a small bowl, combine the mayo, lemon zest, lemon juice, garlic, and salt. Stir until well combined.

TO ASSEMBLE Place the koftas in lettuce cups and add cucumber, tomato, and red onion. Top with the lemon-garlic aioli and serve.

from
MY KITCHEN
to YOURS

I keep my kofta wraps Whole30-approved by serving mine in lettuce cups; however, my kiddos enjoy theirs in pita pockets!

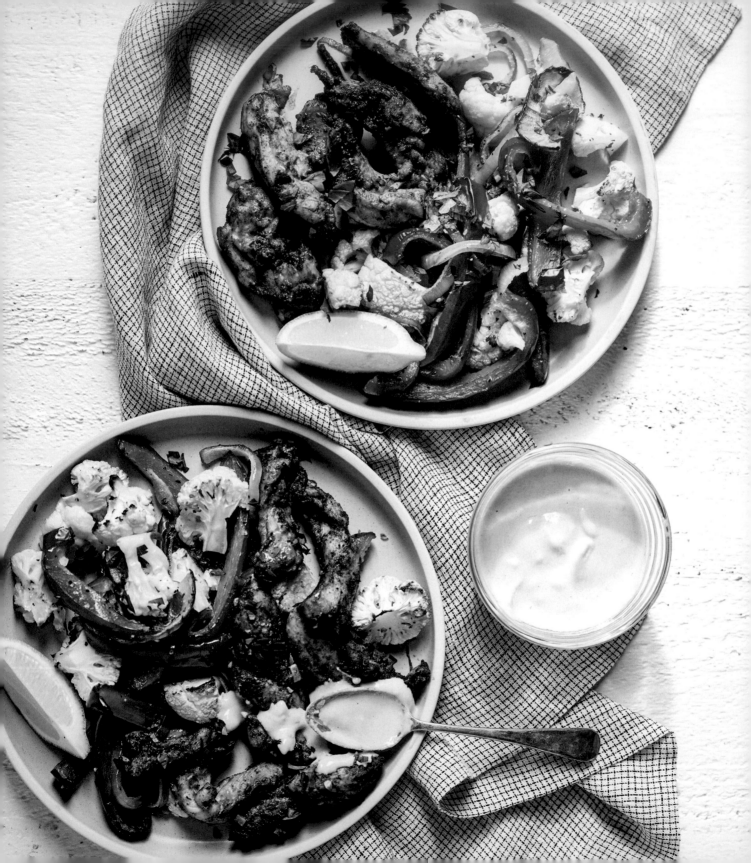

SHEET-PAN CHICKEN SHAWARMA *with* LEMON-TAHINI DRIZZLE

SERVES 6

→ GLUTEN-FREE

→ DAIRY-FREE

→ PALEO

→ WHOLE30 IF MODIFIED

→ GRAIN-FREE

Total time: 45 MINUTES

There isn't a busy weeknight that doesn't love a good sheet-pan meal. Throw it all on a sheet pan, toss it in the oven, and let it cook away while you tend to other important business . . . . It's just too good to be true. This Middle Eastern–inspired feast is a total keeper and is going to have you hooked at first bite. The whole meal comes together in less than 45 minutes and is packed with some of my favorite warming spices, which are also used a lot in Middle Eastern cuisine, like cumin, cinnamon, and paprika—making this meal rich and decadent.

Preheat the oven to 400°F and line 2 large rimmed baking sheets with parchment paper.

MAKE THE CHICKEN Place the sliced chicken in a large bowl with the olive oil, garlic, salt, black pepper, cayenne pepper, paprika, cumin, cinnamon, lemon zest, and lemon juice. Toss to coat evenly and set aside.

MAKE THE VEGGIES On one of the prepared baking sheets, place the red onion, red bell pepper, and cauliflower florets. Add the olive oil, salt, pepper, and oregano. Toss to coat until the veggies are evenly coated.

On the other prepared baking sheet, spread the chicken mixture in a single, even layer.

{ continued }

FOR THE CHICKEN

2 pounds boneless, skinless chicken thighs, trimmed and sliced ½-inch thick

1 tablespoon extra virgin olive oil

2 cloves garlic, minced

1 teaspoon kosher salt

¾ teaspoon freshly ground black pepper

¼ teaspoon cayenne pepper

1 teaspoon paprika

1 teaspoon ground cumin

¼ teaspoon ground cinnamon

Grated zest of ½ lemon (1 teaspoon)

1 tablespoon fresh lemon juice (½ lemon)

FOR THE VEGGIES
(on following page)

FOR THE VEGGIES

- 1½ cups red onion, sliced (¾ medium)
- 2 medium red bell peppers, cut in ¼-inch slices (3 cups)
- 4 cups cauliflower florets (1 small head)
- 2 tablespoons extra virgin olive oil
- ½ teaspoon kosher salt
- ¼ teaspoon freshly ground black pepper
- 1 teaspoon dried oregano

FOR THE LEMON-TAHINI DRIZZLE

- 2 tablespoons tahini
- 2 tablespoons olive oil
- 2 tablespoons fresh lemon juice (1 lemon)
- 2 tablespoons warm water
- 1 clove garlic, minced
- ½ teaspoon honey (optional; omit for Whole30)

Chopped fresh flat-leaf parsley leaves, for serving

- 1 lemon, cut into wedges, for serving

Transfer both of the sheets to the oven and bake for 20 to 25 minutes, until the chicken is cooked through and the veggies are just tender.

MAKE THE DRIZZLE Meanwhile, in a small jar or container, combine all the drizzle ingredients. Shake until well combined and set aside until ready to serve.

When the chicken is done, remove the chicken and veggies from the oven. Distribute the veggies and chicken onto six plates, garnish with chopped parsley, and drizzle with the tahini drizzle. Serve with a wedge of lemon.

from
MY KITCHEN
to YOURS

If you have leftover lemon-tahini drizzle, it will likely harden when you store it in the fridge. To thin it for serving, simply add about 1 tablespoon of warm water and shake it.

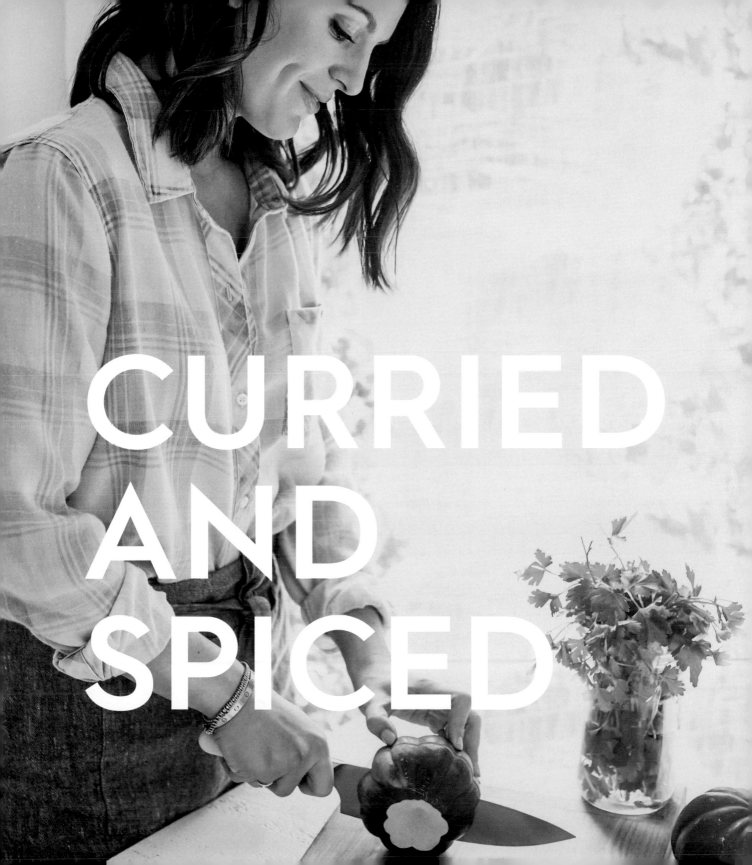

CURRIED
AND
SPICED

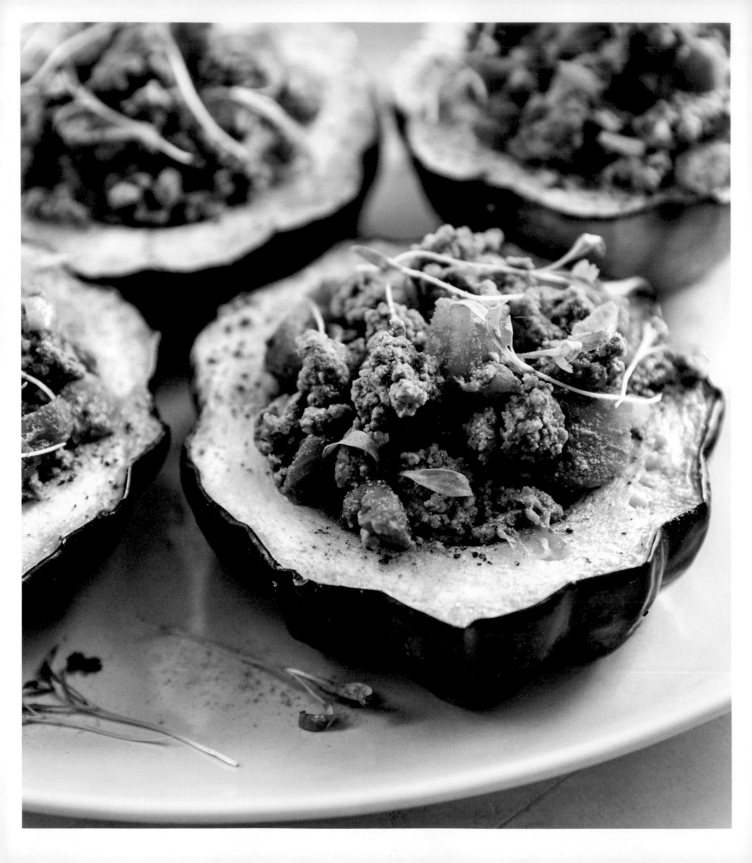

CURRIED BEEF-STUFFED ACORN SQUASH

SERVES 4

→ GLUTEN-FREE

→ DAIRY-FREE

→ PALEO

→ WHOLE30

→ GRAIN-FREE

Total time: 30 MINUTES

This recipe is one of my favorites, and that's saying a lot because it's kinda like picking a favorite child. I'm always excited about how quickly this dish comes together and yet has so many complex layers of flavor. The spiced curried beef combined with the sweet acorn squash really is a match made in heaven.

MAKE THE SQUASH Preheat the oven to 375°F and line a large baking sheet with parchment paper.

Trim the ends of the squash, halve them crosswise, and scoop out the seeds. Place the squash cut-side up on the baking sheet and brush the flesh with olive oil to evenly coat. Sprinkle with salt, pepper, and cinnamon. Bake until the flesh of the squash is fork-tender, 30 to 35 minutes.

MAKE THE CURRIED BEEF Heat the olive oil in a large skillet over medium-high heat until it shimmers. Add the ground beef, onion, salt, and pepper and cook, breaking up the meat with the back of a spoon, until it is no longer pink, 6 to 7 minutes. Drain off any excess fat.

Reduce the heat to medium and add the ginger and garlic. Cook until the garlic is fragrant, 1 to 2 minutes. Add the drained diced tomatoes, curry powder, cumin, and cayenne pepper and stir to combine. Pour in the broth and cook until it reduces, about 3 minutes. Taste and add more salt and/or cayenne, if desired. Remove the pan from the heat, cover, and keep warm until the squash are ready.

Divide the meat mixture between the squash, stuffing the meat in each cavity. Top each with the cilantro and serve.

FOR THE ACORN SQUASH

- 2 medium-size acorn squash
- 2 tablespoons extra virgin olive oil
- ½ teaspoon kosher salt
- ¼ teaspoon freshly ground black pepper
- ¼ teaspoon ground cinnamon

FOR THE CURRIED BEEF

- 1 tablespoon extra virgin olive oil
- 1 pound ground beef (95 percent lean)
- ½ finely diced yellow onion (1 cup)
- ½ teaspoon kosher salt
- ¼ teaspoon freshly ground black pepper
- 1 (½-inch) piece fresh ginger, finely grated
- 2 garlic cloves, minced
- 1 (14.5-ounce) can diced tomatoes, drained
- 1 tablespoon curry powder
- ½ teaspoon ground cumin
- ¼ teaspoon cayenne pepper
- ¼ cup low-sodium vegetable or beef broth
- 2 tablespoons fresh cilantro micro greens, for serving

SERVES 4

→ GLUTEN-FREE

→ DAIRY-FREE

→ PALEO

→ WHOLE30

→ GRAIN-FREE

Total time: 4 TO 6 HOURS
(ABOUT 1 HOUR USING THE
INSTANT POT)

SLOW COOKER CHICKEN TIKKA MASALA

- 2 pounds boneless, skinless chicken breasts, cut into 1-inch cubes
- ¾ cup low-sodium chicken broth
- 2 cups diced yellow onion (1 large)
- 1 (6-ounce) can tomato paste
- 2 tablespoons extra virgin olive oil
- 4 garlic cloves, minced
- 1 (1-inch) piece fresh ginger, finely grated
- 1 tablespoon curry powder
- 1½ teaspoons kosher salt
- 1 teaspoon freshly ground black pepper
- 1 teaspoon ground turmeric
- 1 teaspoon ground cumin
- 1 teaspoon paprika
- ½ teaspoon cayenne pepper (adjust according to your heat preference)
- ½ teaspoon ground cinnamon
- 1 bay leaf
- 1 (13-ounce) can unsweetened full-fat coconut milk (shaken to combine well)
- 2 tablespoons arrowroot starch
- 1 tablespoon fresh lemon juice (½ lemon)
  Prepared Cauliflower Rice (page 282) or basmati rice (optional)
- ¼ cup fresh cilantro leaves, for serving

This meal is the golden ticket, y'all! Throw all the ingredients in a slow cooker or Instant Pot (see below), forget all about it, then come home to a delicious, comforting dinner packed with flavor and ready to be served. I mean, does life get any better than that? Nope. I didn't think so.

In a slow cooker, combine the cubed chicken, broth, onion, tomato paste, olive oil, garlic, ginger, curry powder, salt, black pepper, turmeric, cumin, paprika, cayenne pepper, and cinnamon. Stir until well combined. Place the bay leaf on top, cover, and cook on low for 6 hours or on high for 4 hours.

When the cook time is complete, in a medium bowl, whisk together the coconut milk and arrowroot. Add the mixture to the slow cooker with the cooked chicken and stir to combine. Cook on high for an additional 10 minutes, uncovered and stirring occasionally, to thicken. Once the masala has thickened, stir in the lemon juice. Discard the bay leaf.

To serve, fill four bowls with rice (if desired), and divide the masala mixture among the bowls. Garnish with the cilantro and serve.

INSTANT POT METHOD

Combine the chicken, broth, onion, tomato paste, olive oil, garlic, ginger, curry powder, salt, black pepper, turmeric,

{ continued }

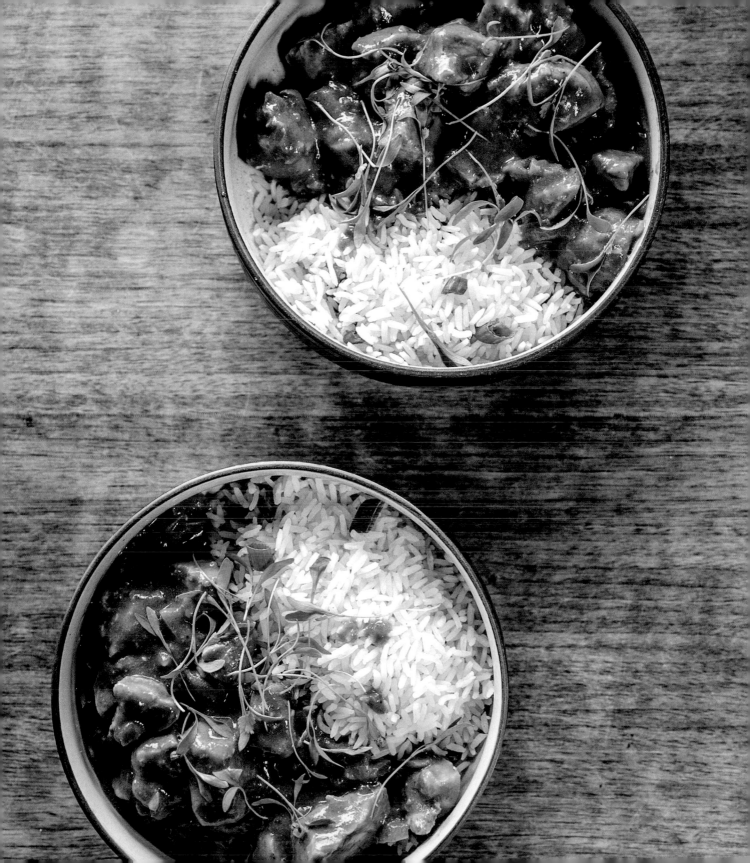

cumin, paprika, cayenne pepper, and cinnamon in the Instant Pot. Stir well. Place the bay leaf on top, cover and seal. Press the poultry button and increase time to 20 minutes.

When cook time is complete, release the pressure manually by carefully turning the valve and opening the Instant Pot. Discard the bay leaf. Turn on the sauté function. In a medium bowl, whisk together the coconut milk and arrowroot starch. Add the mixture to the Instant Pot with the cooked chicken and let simmer until the sauce has thickened, about 10 more minutes.

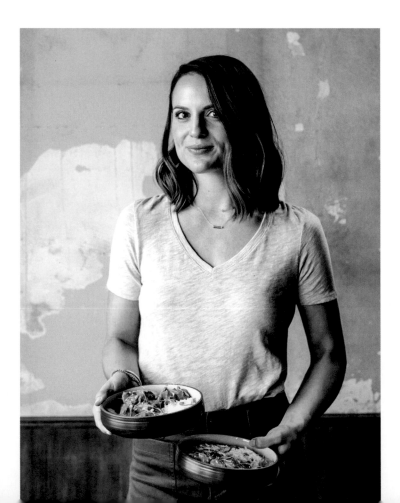

TANDOORI CHICKEN BURGERS *with* CUMIN AIOLI *and* CRISPY OKRA FRIES

SERVES 6
→ GLUTEN-FREE
→ DAIRY-FREE
→ PALEO
→ WHOLE30
→ GRAIN-FREE
Total time: 40 MINUTES

Tandoori chicken is one of those Indian dishes that everyone loves, me included. However, to cook an authentic tandoori chicken, you need a bell-shaped wood-fired clay oven, or tandoor (hence the name). If you own one, that is awesome and I am jealous. But if you don't, I've developed a recipe that borrows traditional tandoor flavors like paprika, cumin, ginger, and garlic and uses them to spice up some easy-peasy chicken burgers instead, along with a cumin-scented aioli for good measure. When I first made this recipe, my husband had three in one sitting! Since then, this recipe has been requested *a lot*. The flavors are exquisite, and the really good news? These aren't spicy, so kids love them, too. Pair the burgers with some simple Crispy Okra Fries and you have yourself one amazing weeknight meal.

MAKE THE AIOLI In a small bowl or jar, combine the mayo, garlic, lemon juice, cumin, and salt and stir to combine. Taste and adjust the seasoning with more salt, if desired. Refrigerate until ready to serve.

MAKE THE CHICKEN BURGERS In a large bowl, combine the chicken, red onion, egg, curry powder, cumin, salt, paprika, coriander, garlic powder, ginger, and pepper. Use your hands to mix until just combined.

Use a measuring cup to scoop out ½ cup of the meat mixture. Using your hands, form it into a round hamburger patty. Transfer

{ continued }

FOR THE CUMIN AIOLI
- ½ cup homemade mayo (page 281)
- 2 garlic cloves, minced
- 2 tablespoons fresh lemon juice (1 lemon)
- 1 teaspoon ground cumin
- ½ teaspoon kosher salt

FOR THE CHICKEN BURGERS
- 2 pounds ground chicken thighs
- ½ cup finely diced red onion (½ medium)
- 1 large egg, beaten
- 2 teaspoons curry powder
- 1 teaspoon ground cumin
- 1 teaspoon kosher salt
- ½ teaspoon paprika
- ½ teaspoon ground coriander
- ½ teaspoon garlic powder
- ½ teaspoon ground ginger
- ½ teaspoon freshly ground black pepper
- 2 tablespoons avocado oil

TO ASSEMBLE
(on following page)

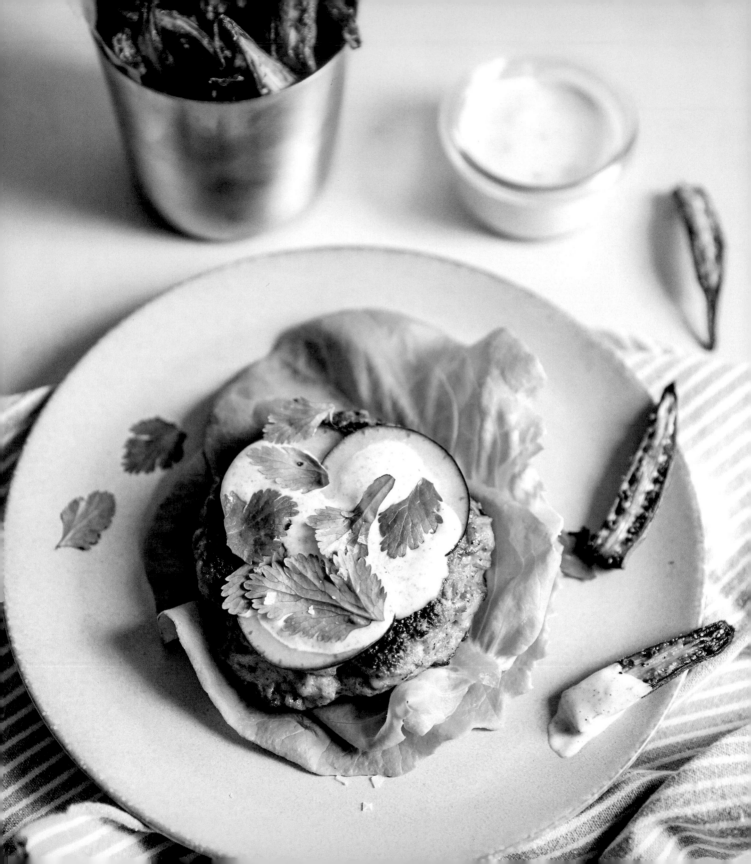

TO ASSEMBLE

Butter lettuce leaves or 6 buns

½ cucumber, thinly sliced

¼ cup fresh cilantro leaves

Crispy Okra Fries (recipe follows)

to a large parchment paper–lined plate and repeat with the remaining mixture, until 6 patties are formed.

In a large skillet (preferably cast-iron), heat the avocado oil over medium-high heat. When the oil is hot but not yet smoking, carefully place the patties in the skillet, being careful not to overcrowd the pan. You will likely need to do this in 2 batches. Reduce the heat to medium and sear the patties on each side until golden brown and cooked through, 4 to 5 minutes per side. Transfer the cooked burgers to a paper towel–lined plate and repeat with the remaining burgers.

TO ASSEMBLE Wrap each burger in lettuce leaves or set on a bun. Top with the sliced cucumbers, cilantro, and a dollop of the aioli. Serve with okra fries (if desired) and aioli for dipping.

CRISPY OKRA FRIES

TOTAL TIME: 40 minutes

1 pound fresh okra, tops removed and sliced lengthwise

2 tablespoons avocado oil

½ teaspoon garlic powder

1 teaspoon kosher salt

½ teaspoon freshly ground black pepper

Preheat the oven to 375°F. Top a large baking sheet with a wire rack and set aside.

In a large bowl, combine the sliced okra with the avocado oil, garlic powder, salt, and pepper. Toss to evenly coat.

Arrange the okra on top of the wire rack in a single layer. (Do not overcrowd the pan or let any pieces overlap, or the okra will not crisp up. You may need to use two baking sheets.) Roast for 25 to 30 minutes, until the okra is golden brown and crispy. Serve hot.

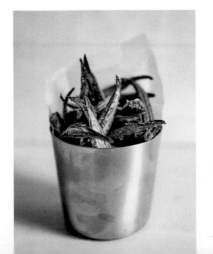

SERVES 2

→ GLUTEN-FREE

→ DAIRY-FREE

→ PALEO

→ WHOLE30

→ GRAIN-FREE

Total time: 30 MINUTES

GARAM MASALA-RUBBED LAMB CHOPS *with a* SIMPLE FENNEL *and* ARUGULA SALAD

FOR THE LAMB CHOPS

8 lamb rib chops (about 2 pounds)

1 teaspoon kosher salt

½ teaspoon freshly ground black pepper

¼ cup plus 1 tablespoon extra virgin olive oil

2 cloves garlic, minced

1½ teaspoons garam marsala

FOR THE FENNEL AND ARUGULA SALAD

1 small fennel bulb

3 cups baby arugula

2 tablespoons extra virgin olive oil

2 tablespoons fresh lemon juice (1 lemon)

½ teaspoon kosher salt

¼ teaspoon freshly ground black pepper

This recipe is what I like to call a magic trick. You give little to no effort to get a restaurant-quality, healthy dinner on the table. Lamb chops look fancy (and they kind of are) but take only minutes to sear on each side, and the end result is simply fantastic. I marinate my lamb in a garam masala spice blend. It's certainly not spicy, but the combination of spices like cinnamon, cloves, cumin, and coriander within the garam masala give it a warm, delicious flavor. Served alongside a fresh and crisp fennel and arugula salad, dinner will be ready in no time and absolutely delightful.

MARINATE THE LAMB CHOPS Place the lamb chops in a shallow bowl and season with salt and pepper. In a small bowl, combine ¼ cup olive oil, the minced garlic, and garam masala. Whisk to combine, then pour over the lamb chops and toss to coat evenly. Set aside and let marinate at room temperature for 15 minutes while you prepare your salad.

MAKE THE SALAD Trim and discard the outer layers and fronds from the fennel. Slice it paper thin using a mandoline or knife and place in a large bowl with the baby arugula. Set aside.

{ continued }

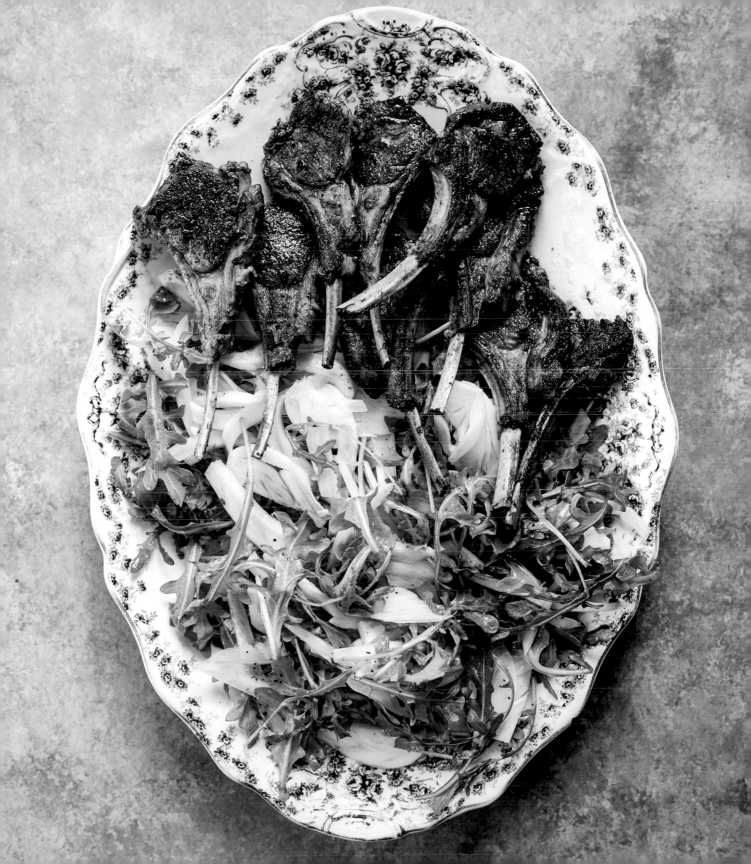

In a small bowl, whisk together the olive oil, lemon juice, salt, and pepper. Set aside.

COOK THE LAMB CHOPS After the ribs have marinated, in a large skillet, heat the remaining 1 tablespoon olive oil over medium-high heat until shimmering. Working in batches, cook the lamb chops in the pan until brown and crusty, 2 to 3 minutes per side for medium-rare. Transfer the lamb to a cutting board or platter and let rest for 5 to 10 minutes before serving.

After the chops have rested and immediately before serving, pour the dressing over the salad and toss to coat evenly. Divide the salad between two plates and top with the seared lamb chops.

CURRIED TUNA CAKES *with* LEMONY ASPARAGUS

SERVES 4

→ GLUTEN-FREE

→ DAIRY-FREE

→ PALEO

→ WHOLE30

→ GRAIN-FREE

Total time: 35 MINUTES

There are many things in life that I learned from my mother. She taught me to be a great and loyal friend, a loving wife, a patient mother, a voting citizen, and . . . she taught me that there are about 1 million ways to use a can of tuna. No joke! My mom has always worked full time and was always on the run, yet still managed to make herself and our family healthy meals. I was fascinated by the many ways she could use a can of tuna: on salads, in sandwiches, in pasta . . . I mean, the possibilities were really endless. My sister and I laugh about it all the time because we now find ourselves, in our adult lives, doing the same. For example, check out this recipe. I've seriously jazzed up canned tuna by adding some delicious flavor, forming it into patties, and pan-searing them on the stove top. Topped with a little curried mayo, it's just *so good* and *so easy*.

MAKE THE CURRIED MAYO Combine all of the mayo ingredients in a small bowl and stir to combine. Refrigerate until ready to serve.

MAKE THE TUNA CAKES Place the drained tuna in a large bowl and using the back of a fork, break up the fish. Add the egg, bell pepper, green onions, curry powder, mayo, almond flour, raisins, salt, and pepper. Using a fork, mix until well combined.

Using a ¼-cup measuring cup, scoop out the mixture, then form into round patties. Continue until all the mixture is used.

In a large skillet, heat the avocado oil over medium-high heat and swirl the pan to evenly coat.

{ continued }

FOR THE CURRIED MAYO

¼ cup homemade mayo (page 281)

¼ teaspoon kosher salt

¼ teaspoon curry powder

1 tablespoon fresh lemon juice (½ lemon)

FOR THE TUNA CAKES

2 (5-ounce) cans of tuna (no salt added, drained)

1 large egg

¼ cup finely diced red bell pepper (¼ small)

¼ cup thinly sliced green onions (white and green parts; about 2)

1 teaspoon curry powder

2 tablespoons homemade mayo (page 281)

¼ cup almond flour

2 tablespoons golden raisins, loosely chopped

½ teaspoon kosher salt

¼ teaspoon freshly ground black pepper

2 tablespoons avocado oil

Fresh chopped parsley, for serving

Lemony Asparagus (recipe follows)

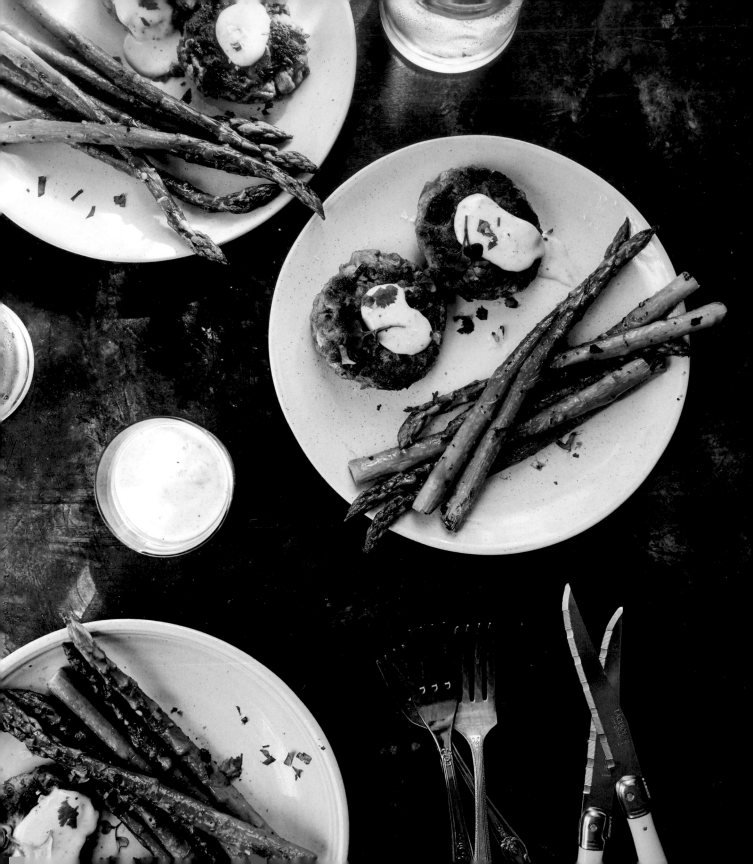

When the oil is hot, use a spatula to carefully lay the cakes into the oil and let fry until golden brown, about 3 minutes. Using a spatula, carefully flip and continue to cook on the other side until golden brown, 2 to 3 more minutes.

Transfer the patties onto a plate lined with paper towels. Serve with curried mayo, chopped parsley, and lemony asparagus.

LEMONY ASPARAGUS

TOTAL TIME: 12 minutes

- 1 bunch asparagus, woody ends trimmed
- 1 tablespoon extra virgin olive oil
- 2 cloves garlic, minced
- ¼ teaspoon crushed red pepper
- Grated zest of ½ lemon (1½ teaspoons)
- ½ teaspoon kosher salt
- ½ teaspoon freshly ground black pepper
- 1 tablespoon fresh lemon juice (½ lemon)

Fill a large skillet three-quarters full with water and bring to a boil. Add the asparagus to boiling water and cook for 3 minutes, then immediately transfer the stalks to a bowl of ice water to stop them from cooking. Drain and set aside.

Drain the water from the skillet and return to the stove top over medium-high heat with the olive oil. When the oil is shimmering, using tongs, transfer the asparagus back to the skillet and add the garlic, crushed red pepper, lemon zest, salt, and pepper.

Cook, tossing occasionally, until the asparagus is tender and lightly golden on the edges, about 4 to 5 minutes. Squeeze the fresh lemon over it and serve immediately.

SERVES 2

→ GLUTEN-FREE

→ DAIRY-FREE

→ PALEO

→ WHOLE30

→ GRAIN-FREE

Total time: 20 MINUTES

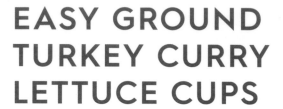

EASY GROUND TURKEY CURRY LETTUCE CUPS

Have you ever caught yourself wishing for more hours in the day? If so, this recipe will help you keep your dinnertime prep short and sweet. Lean ground turkey finished with easy-to-find Indian spices makes for a healthy and filling dish. The warming spices in combination with the sweet golden raisins are a match made in heaven! If you are a curry lover but want to make something using minimal ingredients and less time, this one is perfect for you!

---

2 tablespoons extra virgin olive oil

1 cup finely diced yellow onion (1 medium)

1 pound ground turkey (preferably dark meat)

1 (½-inch) piece fresh ginger, finely grated

2 cloves garlic, minced

½ teaspoon kosher salt, or more to taste

1 teaspoon curry powder

¼ teaspoon cayenne pepper (optional)

¾ cup unsweetened full-fat coconut milk

¼ cup golden raisins

TO ASSEMBLE

½ cup matchstick carrots

8 large butter lettuce leaves

¼ cup fresh cilantro leaves

In a large skillet, heat the oil over medium-high heat until shimmering. Add the onion, ground turkey, ginger, and garlic and cook, breaking up the meat with the back of a spoon, until the turkey is cooked through (no longer pink) and browned, about 5 minutes.

Add the salt, curry powder, and cayenne pepper (if using) and cook, stirring, for 1 more minute.

Add the coconut milk and raisins, stir to combine, and cook until the coconut milk is heated through and coats the meat, 2 to 3 more minutes.

To serve, sprinkle matchstick carrots in the bottom of a lettuce leaf, add a big scoop of the curried turkey, and top it all off with a few cilantro leaves.

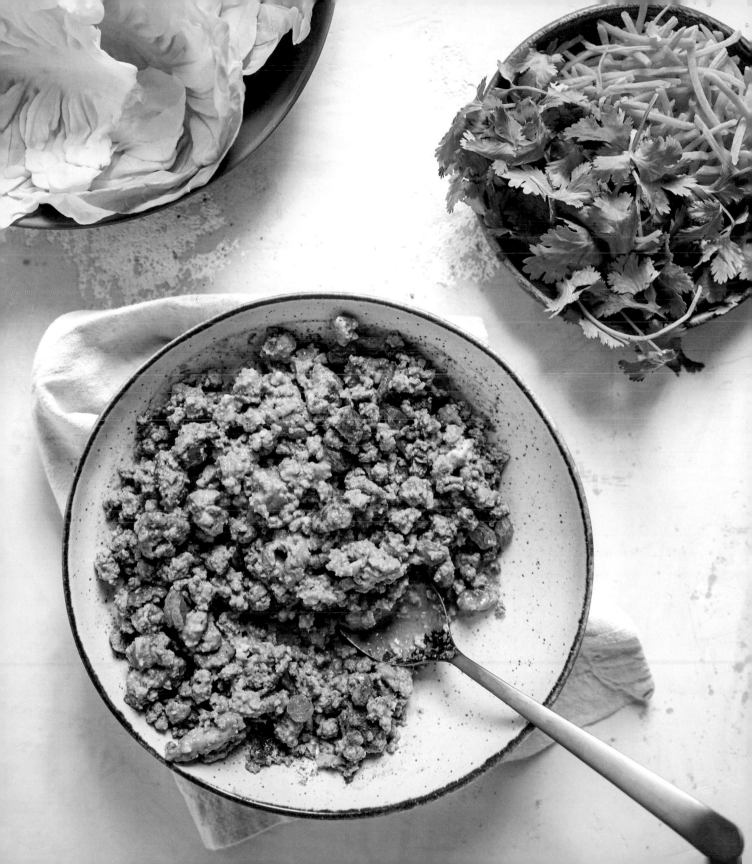

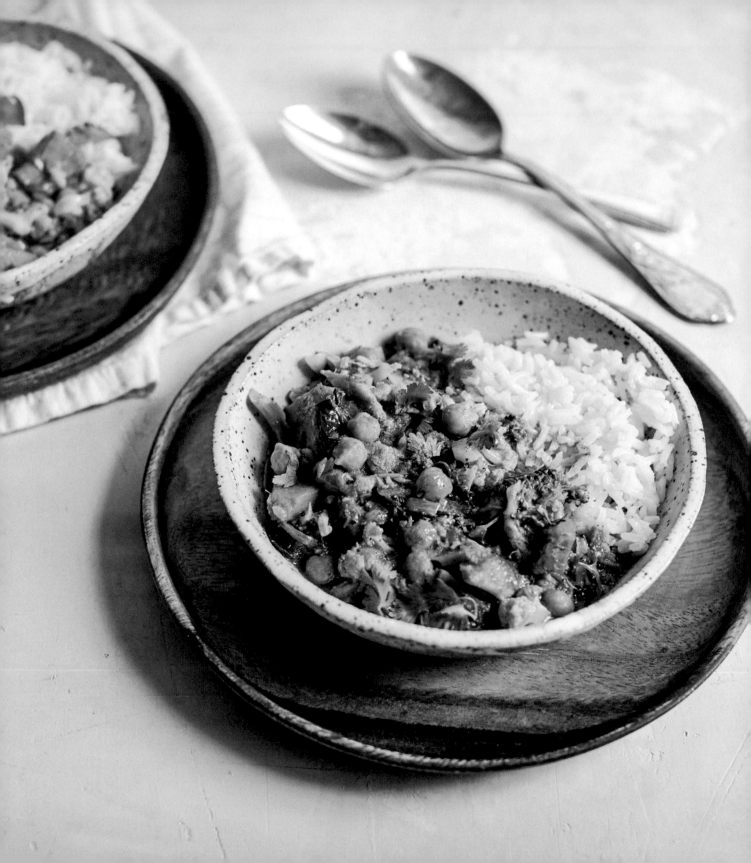

INDIAN-STYLE VEGETABLE CURRY

SERVES 4

→ GLUTEN-FREE

→ DAIRY-FREE

→ PALEO IF MODIFIED

→ WHOLE30 IF MODIFIED

→ GRAIN-FREE

Total time: 40 MINUTES

One of my favorite things about Indian food is how delicious the vegetarian dishes are. I absolutely love the combination of spices that blend together to make fragrant, flavorful sauces that, even without the addition of meat, have such comforting appeal. When I am feeling like I really need to increase my vegetable intake, I cook up this one-pot wonder and immediately feel like I am nourishing my body. Not only because the veggies are so good for me, but also because the spices have their own antioxidant powers, too!

In a Dutch oven or large pot, heat the olive oil over medium heat. Add the shallots and garlic and cook, stirring, until tender, about 2 to 3 minutes. Stir in the tomato paste, cumin, turmeric, curry powder, cinnamon, coriander, ginger, and cayenne pepper. Cook until the spices have toasted and become fragrant, about 2 minutes.

Pour in the coconut milk and broth and stir to combine. Add the cauliflower, broccoli, sweet potato, tomatoes, and salt. Stir to combine and bring to a boil. Once boiling, reduce the heat to a gentle simmer, cover, and let the mixture cook, adding the drained chickpeas 15 minutes into the cooking process. Continue cooking until the vegetables are tender, an additional 10 minutes. Stir in the spinach, lime zest, and lime juice and cook until the spinach is just wilted, about 2 minutes. Serve over prepared rice and sprinkle with cilantro.

2 tablespoons extra virgin olive oil

2 large shallots, finely diced (½ cup)

3 garlic cloves, minced

1 tablespoon tomato paste

2 teaspoons ground cumin

1 teaspoon ground turmeric

1 teaspoon curry powder

1 teaspoon ground cinnamon

½ teaspoon ground coriander

½ teaspoon ground ginger

¼ teaspoon cayenne pepper

1 (13-ounce) can unsweetened full-fat coconut milk

1½ cups vegetable broth

1 small head of cauliflower, cut into florets (about 3 cups)

1 small head of broccoli, cut into florets (about 3 cups)

1 large sweet potato, peeled and cut into 1-inch cubes (about 3 cups)

2 medium tomatoes, seeded and diced

1½ teaspoons kosher salt

1 (15-ounce) can chickpeas, drained and rinsed (omit for Whole30/paleo)

4 cups packed baby spinach

Grated zest of ½ lime

1 tablespoon fresh lime juice

1½ cups cooked basmati rice or Prepared Cauliflower Rice (page 282), for serving

¼ cup fresh cilantro leaves

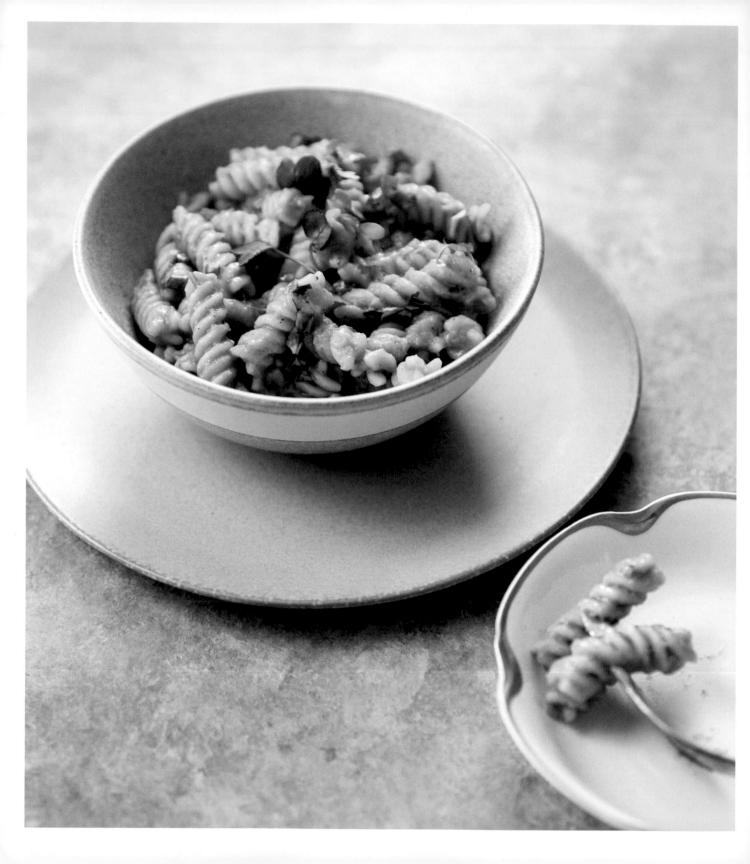

ONE-POT COCONUT CURRY BUTTERNUT SQUASH PASTA

SERVES 4
→ GLUTEN-FREE
→ DAIRY-FREE
Total time: 40 MINUTES

This one-pot coconut curry looks like a grown-up mac 'n' cheese, and it kind of is one—except for the fact that it is dairy-free and is kicked up a notch with Indian-inspired flavors. So maybe we will just say it's mac 'n' cheese's really cool older cousin? Anywho, this pasta has a fantastically silky, creamy, and aromatic coconut curry sauce made from a pureed butternut squash that will really change up your typical weeknight meal.

In a large pot, heat the olive oil over medium heat. Add the shallot and garlic and gently cook until the shallot is tender, about 3 minutes. Increase the heat to medium-high and add the butternut squash, broth, curry powder, salt, black pepper, cumin, cinnamon, and cayenne pepper and bring to a boil. Reduce the heat to a simmer, cover, and cook until the butternut squash is fork-tender, about 15 minutes.

Stir in the coconut milk and use an immersion blender to blend until smooth and creamy. Alternatively, transfer the mixture to a high-powered blender and blend in batches, then return the sauce to the pot. Bring the sauce to a simmer, add the pasta, and cook, uncovered and stirring often, until the pasta is al dente and has absorbed a lot of the sauce, about 15 minutes. Season with salt to taste.

To serve, divide the pasta among 4 serving bowls and sprinkle with the cilantro and red pepper flakes if desired.

2 tablespoons extra virgin olive oil

1 large shallot, finely diced (¼ cup)

2 garlic cloves, minced

1 large butternut squash, peeled and cut into 1-inch cubes (about 4 cups)

2 cups low-sodium chicken or vegetable broth

2 teaspoons curry powder

1 teaspoon kosher salt

½ teaspoon freshly ground black pepper

¼ teaspoon ground cumin

¼ teaspoon ground cinnamon

⅛ teaspoon cayenne pepper

1 (13-ounce) can unsweetened full-fat coconut milk

16 ounces brown rice fusilli pasta (I use Jovial brand)

FOR SERVING

¼ cup roughly chopped fresh cilantro leaves

Crushed red pepper flakes (optional)

SERVES 8

→ GLUTEN-FREE

→ DAIRY-FREE

→ PALEO

→ WHOLE30

→ GRAIN-FREE

Total time: 8 HOURS,
15 MINUTES

CURRIED POT ROAST

A pot roast is the perfect weeknight meal. Requiring a little effort in the morning (or even the night before—thank you, slow cooker!), you come home to dinner ready to be served. And better yet, it fills everybody's belly. Even this unique curried rendition is a family favorite at our house, and one that my kids gladly gobble up.

FOR THE ROAST

- 3 pounds boneless beef chuck roast
- 2 teaspoons kosher salt
- 1 teaspoon freshly ground black pepper
- 3 tablespoons arrowroot starch
- 2 tablespoons extra virgin olive oil
- 1 pound medium-size red potatoes, quartered
- 1 medium yellow onion, halved and cut into ½-inch slices
- 2 medium carrots, cut into 2-inch chunks
- 1 dried bay leaf

FOR THE CURRY SAUCE

- 1 (14.5-ounce) can diced fire-roasted tomatoes
- ½ cup low-sodium beef broth
- 1 (½-inch) piece fresh ginger, finely grated
- 1 tablespoon mustard
- 1 tablespoon apple cider vinegar
- 2 teaspoons curry powder
- 2 garlic cloves
- ½ teaspoon ground cumin
- ½ teaspoon ground turmeric

MAKE THE ROAST Season the roast all over with the salt and pepper.

Pour the arrowroot onto a large plate or shallow bowl, then dredge the roast to coat completely. Shake off any excess arrowroot.

In a large skillet, heat the olive oil over medium-high heat until just smoking. Add the roast and sear until a deep brown crust forms, 3 to 4 minutes on each side. Transfer the browned roast to a slow cooker.

Nestle the potatoes, onion slices, and carrots around the roast and drop in the bay leaf. Set aside.

MAKE THE CURRY SAUCE In a food processor or blender, combine the tomatoes and can juices, broth, ginger, mustard, vinegar, curry powder, garlic, cumin, and turmeric. Blend until smooth.

Pour the sauce over the roast and vegetables. Cover the slow cooker and cook the roast on high for 4 to 6 hours, or on low for 8 to 10 hours, until the roast is fall-apart tender. Discard the bay leaf and serve.

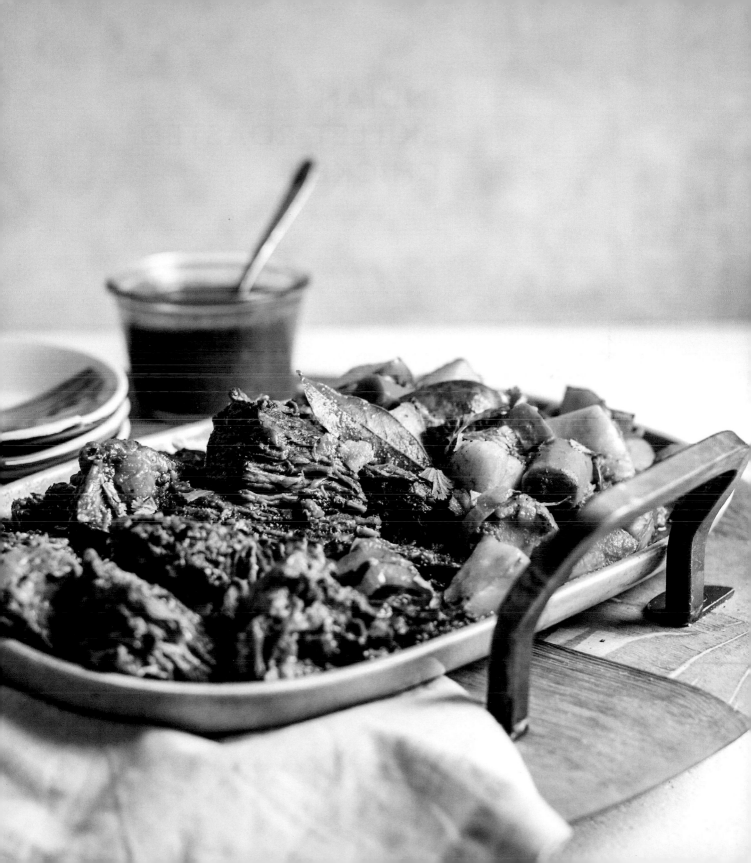

SERVES 4

→ GLUTEN-FREE

→ DAIRY-FREE

→ PALEO

→ WHOLE30

→ GRAIN-FREE

Total time: 55 MINUTES

INDIAN SKILLET-ROASTED CHICKEN

1 (3½- to 4-pound) whole chicken

1 teaspoon curry powder

1 teaspoon paprika

½ teaspoon ground ginger

½ teaspoon garlic powder

½ teaspoon ground cumin

¼ teaspoon cayenne pepper

½ teaspoon ground coriander

¼ teaspoon ground cinnamon

1 teaspoon kosher salt plus more to taste

½ teaspoon freshly ground black pepper plus more to taste

⅓ cup plus 2 tablespoons extra virgin olive oil

1 small head of cauliflower, cut into 1-inch florets

2 large carrots, cut into 2-inch chunks

1 medium yellow onion, halved and cut into ¼-inch slices

½ lemon, cut into ¼-inch slices

½ cup low-sodium chicken broth

¼ cup fresh cilantro leaves, for serving

Have you ever spatchcocked a chicken? Yeah, I know, I giggle when I see that word too! Aside from its silly sounding name, let me just tell you that it is *the way* to roast your chicken. By removing the backbone your bird will cook more evenly, more quickly, and with even crispier skin! (All it takes is a good pair of poultry shears, though your butcher can do it for you, too.) This rendition of classic roasted chicken won't just have you swooning over how much easier it is to achieve perfection— you'll also be *ooh*ing and *aah*ing over how flavorful it is thanks to an Indian-inspired spice rub. The smells coming from your kitchen will have the whole family sneaking in to ask you "What's for dinner?!"

Preheat the oven to 450°F.

Place the chicken breast-side down. Using sturdy kitchen shears or poultry shears, cut up along each side of the backbone to remove it, cutting through the ribs as you go. Discard the backbone.

Flip the chicken over and open it like a book. Press firmly on the breastbone with the heel of your hand to flatten.

Rinse the chicken, inside and out, and pat until dry.

In a medium bowl, combine the curry powder, paprika, ginger, garlic powder, cumin, cayenne pepper, coriander, cinnamon, salt, and black pepper. Pour in ⅓ cup of the olive oil and whisk until there are no clumps. Set aside.

{ continued }

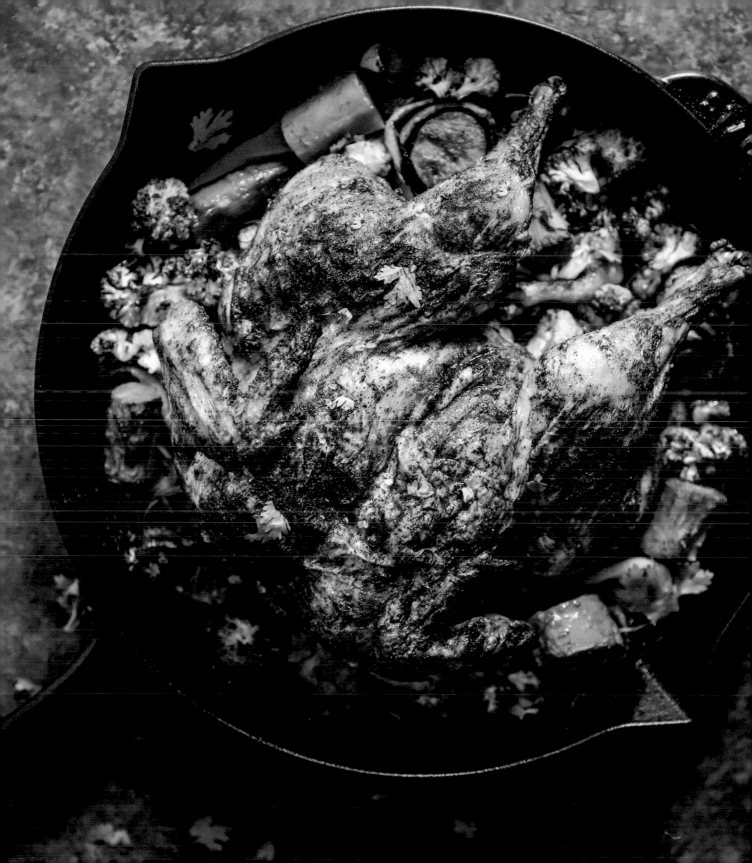

In the bottom of a large skillet or roasting pan, combine the cauliflower, carrots, onion, and lemon slices. Drizzle with the remaining 2 tablespoons olive oil and sprinkle with a little salt and pepper. Toss to coat. Place the butterflied chicken on top of the vegetables skin-side down and brush with about half of the spice rub. Turn the chicken skin-side up, pat the skin dry with paper towels, and brush the remaining spice mixture over the top. Transfer the pan to the oven to roast for 30 minutes.

After roasting for 30 minutes, remove the chicken from the oven but keep the oven on. Pour the broth into the pan, not on top of the chicken, and roast for another 10 to 15 minutes, until a meat thermometer inserted into the thickest part of the breast registers 155 to 160°F.

Carefully tent the chicken with aluminum foil and let rest for 10 to 15 minutes. Quarter the chicken and sprinkle it with a pinch of salt and the cilantro. Serve hot with the pan juices and vegetables.

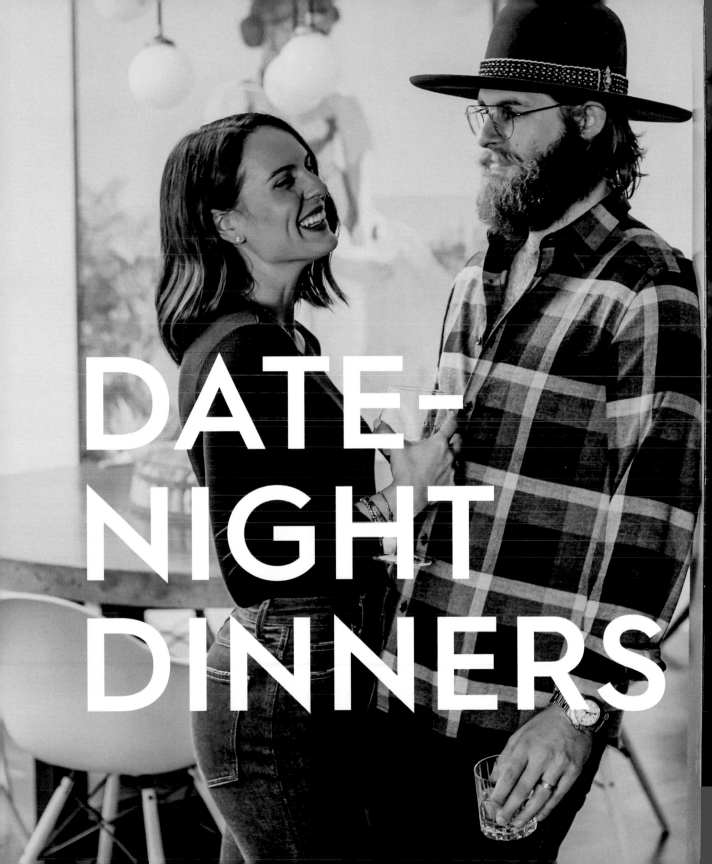

DATE-NIGHT DINNERS

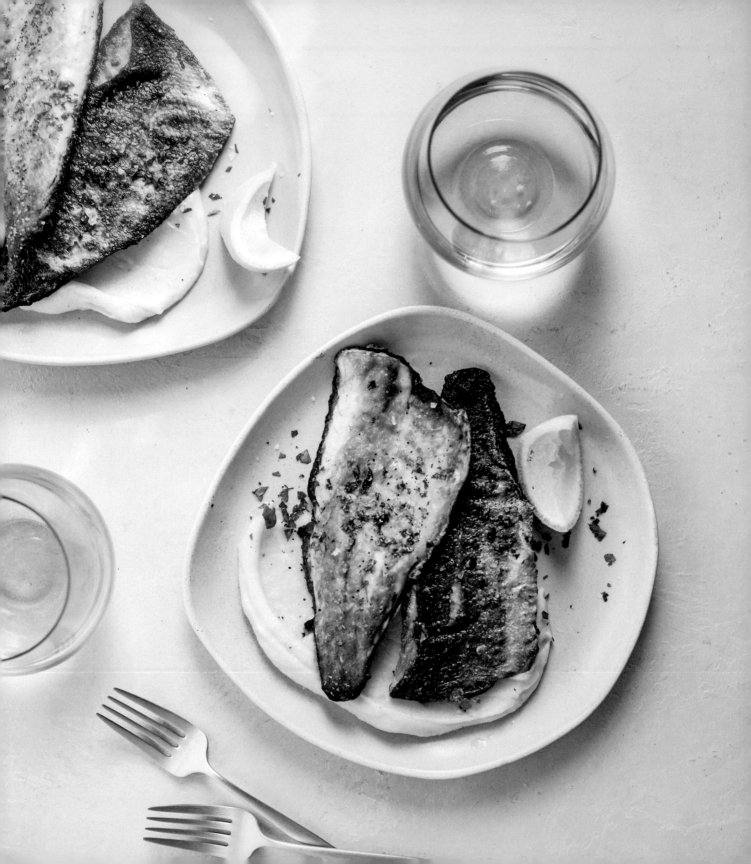

CRISPY-SKINNED BRANZINO *with* PARSNIP PUREE

SERVES 2
→ GLUTEN-FREE
→ DAIRY-FREE
→ PALEO
→ WHOLE30
→ GRAIN-FREE
Total time: 35 MINUTES

Branzino is one of my favorite fish. Its flavor is clean, sweet, fresh, and plays particularly well with other ingredients, which in this case is parsnips that have been blended into a creamy puree with coconut milk, garlic, and thyme. I also love that you can get the skin nice and crispy. My secret technique is to first blot the skin dry and then give it an hour in the fridge to dry out a bit further. (Though you could just blot and cook if you're short on time!) It's a super-easy date-night dish that tastes like a five-star restaurant entrée.

It can sometimes be tricky to find branzino that's portioned into fillets (it's usually sold as the whole fish), but just ask the fishmonger at your grocery store to portion it for you. Then all that stands between you and your date thinking you're an award-winning chef is following this incredibly simple recipe!

Place the fish fillets skin-side up on a baking sheet or plate. Blot the skin dry with a paper towel. Refrigerate the fish, uncovered, for 1 hour to dry out the skin a bit more. (This step is not required; however, it leads to a much crispier skin if you have the time).

In a medium saucepan over high heat, combine the parsnips and chicken broth. Bring to a boil then reduce the heat to a simmer. Cook until the parsnips are fork-tender, about 15 minutes.

4 branzino fillets (about 6 ounces each) (see Headnote)

4 cups parsnips, peeled and cut into 1-inch cubes (about 1 pound parsnips)

2 cups low-sodium chicken broth

¼ cup unsweetened full-fat coconut milk

2 garlic cloves

½ teaspoon dried thyme

½ teaspoon kosher salt, or more to taste

¼ teaspoon freshly ground black pepper, or more to taste

2 tablespoons extra virgin olive oil

1 tablespoon finely chopped fresh flat-leaf parsley leaves, for serving

1 lemon, cut into wedges, for serving

{ continued }

Transfer the parsnips and remaining cooking broth to a blender or food processor. Add the coconut milk, garlic, thyme, salt, and pepper and blend until smooth. Set aside and cover to keep warm.

In a large skillet, heat the olive oil over medium-high heat. Place the fish fillets in the pan, skin-side down and flatten them with the back of a spatula to keep the skin from curling up during the first few minutes of cooking. Cook, pressing occasionally with the spatula, until the fish is nearly opaque and cooked through, with only a small raw area on the very top, about 3 minutes. Flip the fish and remove the skillet from the heat. Let the fish finish cooking and brown in the hot skillet, about 1 more minute.

Divide the parsnip puree between two plates. Place the fish on top, skin-side up. Sprinkle the skin with a pinch of salt, parsley, and serve with lemon wedges.

SHEET PAN RACK *of* LAMB *with* POTATOES *and* MINT CHIMICHURRI

SERVES 2
➔ GLUTEN-FREE
➔ DAIRY-FREE
➔ PALEO
➔ WHOLE30
➔ GRAIN-FREE
Total time: 45 MINUTES

Even though it would be hard for my husband to tell you which dish of mine is his absolute favorite (there's a lot to choose from!), he could easily tell you which gets requested the most: my mint chimichurri. Any time we have guests over and are grilling out in the backyard, it's essential that I make this vibrant, fresh sauce to go with *all* the things. Seriously, it's amazing with pretty much anything—steak, chicken, fish, seafood, veggies—you name it. Since I know my hubby loves it so much, it only made sense that it would become part of this stand-by date-night dish. I highly recommend roasting a fancy-schmancy rack of lamb for your sweetie and topping it with this chimichurri sauce.

MAKE THE CHIMICHURRI In a food processor or blender, combine the mint, parsley, garlic, vinegar, red pepper flakes, salt, and black pepper and pulse until the mixture is finely chopped. Place the mixture into a small bowl and, while whisking, slowly drizzle the olive oil until well combined. Set aside.

MAKE THE LAMB AND POTATOES Preheat the oven to 425°F. Line a large rimmed baking sheet with parchment paper and set aside.

In a medium bowl, whisk together ½ cup of the olive oil, the mustard, garlic, salt, and pepper.

FOR THE MINT CHIMICHURRI
- 1 cup packed fresh mint leaves
- 1 cup packed fresh flat-leaf parsley leaves
- 2 garlic cloves
- ¼ cup red wine vinegar
- ¼ teaspoon crushed red pepper flakes
- ½ teaspoon kosher salt
- ¼ teaspoon freshly ground black pepper
- ½ cup extra virgin olive oil

FOR THE LAMB AND POTATOES
- ½ cup plus 1 tablespoon extra virgin olive oil
- 2 tablespoons mustard
- 2 garlic cloves, minced
- 1 teaspoon kosher salt
- ½ teaspoon freshly ground black pepper
- 1 pound medium-size red potatoes, quartered
- 1 (1½ to 2-pound) rack of lamb, "frenched" (ask your butcher!)

{ continued }

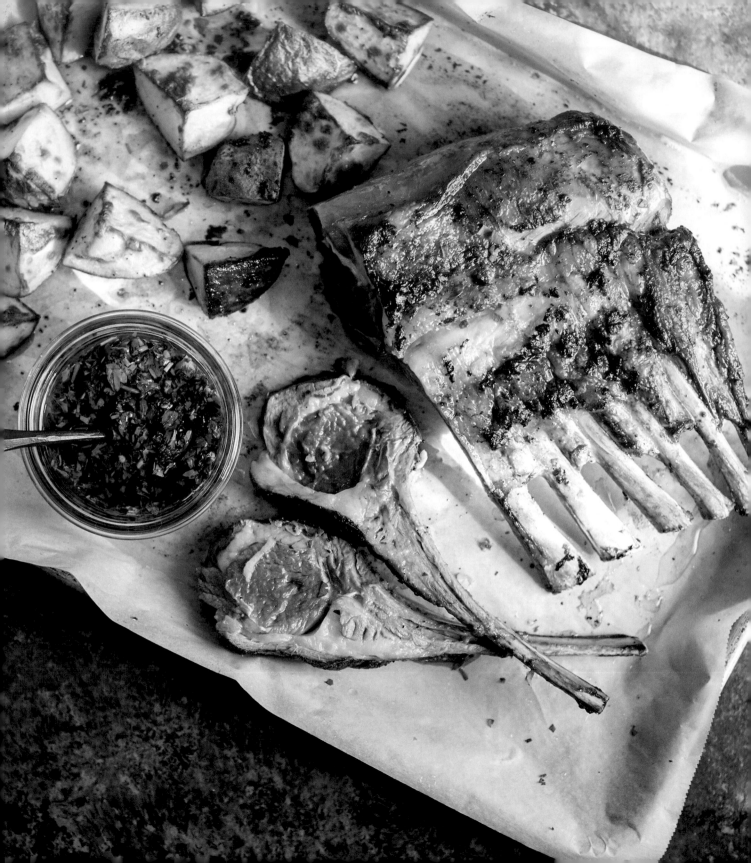

Arrange the potatoes in a single layer on the prepared baking sheet. Pour half of the mustard mixture over the potatoes and toss to evenly coat. Roast for 10 minutes, just to get the potatoes slightly cooked before adding the rack of lamb. Remove the potatoes from the oven but keep the oven on.

Pour the remaining mustard mixture over the rack of lamb and use your hands to rub it evenly over the meat.

In a large skillet, heat the remaining 1 tablespoon olive oil over medium-high heat. When shimmering, carefully place the lamb in the pan fat-side down (ribs curving up) and sear until golden brown, 3 to 4 minutes.

Push the partially roasted potatoes to the outer edges of the sheet pan, making room in the center. Place the lamb in the center, ribs curved down, and roast until the lamb registers 130°F on a meat thermometer for medium-rare, 15 to 20 minutes, depending how thick the lamb is.

Remove the lamb from the oven. Transfer the rack of lamb to a cutting board and cover it with aluminum foil. Allow the lamb to rest for 10 minutes to let the juices settle before slicing between the ribs. Serve with the potatoes and drizzle with the chimichurri.

SERVES 2

→ GLUTEN-FREE IF MODIFIED

→ DAIRY-FREE

Total time: 30 MINUTES

LINGUINE *with* CLAMS, CHILES, *and* SALAMI

1 tablespoon plus ½ teaspoon kosher salt

8 ounces dried pasta, preferably linguine (use gluten-free pasta to modify)

2 tablespoons extra virgin olive oil

2½ ounces dried Italian salami, casing removed, quartered lengthwise, and cut crosswise into ¼-inch slices

3 garlic cloves, thinly sliced

1 Fresno chile, seeded and thinly sliced crosswise (or ½ teaspoon crushed red pepper flakes)

⅓ cup dry white wine

1½ pounds littleneck clams, scrubbed clean

1 (6.5-ounce) can chopped clams, undrained

¼ teaspoon freshly ground black pepper

¼ cup chopped fresh flat-leaf parsley leaves

2 tablespoons fresh lemon juice (1 lemon)

Freshly grated Parmesan, for serving (optional, omit for dairy-free)

To me, nothing is more romantic than a bowl of pasta. And if pasta is my love language, then this dish is definitely the key to my heart. I've taken classic linguine with clams and given it my own spin, spicing things up for date night with salami and Fresno chiles. If you love big, bold flavors like me, you'll just fall in love all over again when you share this dish.

Bring a large pot of water to a boil. Once boiling, salt the water with 1 tablespoon of the salt and add the pasta. Cook according to the package instructions until al dente. Reserve ¼ cup of the pasta water, then drain the pasta and set aside.

In the same pot, heat the olive oil over medium heat until it shimmers. Add the salami, garlic, and chile and cook, stirring, until the garlic is golden and the chiles are tender, about 2 minutes. Raise the heat to medium-high and add the wine. Cook, stirring, until the wine reduces by half, about 2 minutes.

Add the clams and the canned clams and its juices. Stir to combine, cover, and cook until the clams open, about 6 minutes, giving the pot a gentle shake every so often during the process to help the clams cook evenly. Discard any unopened clams.

Return the pasta to the pot and add the remaining ½ teaspoon salt and the pepper. Using tongs, gently toss the pasta in the liquid until evenly coated. Add the parsley and lemon juice and toss once more. Add the remaining ¼ cup of reserved pasta water and continue cooking until the liquid reduces by half and the pasta has a nice light and creamy sauce. Adjust the seasoning with more salt if desired and top with Parmesan, if using. Serve immediately.

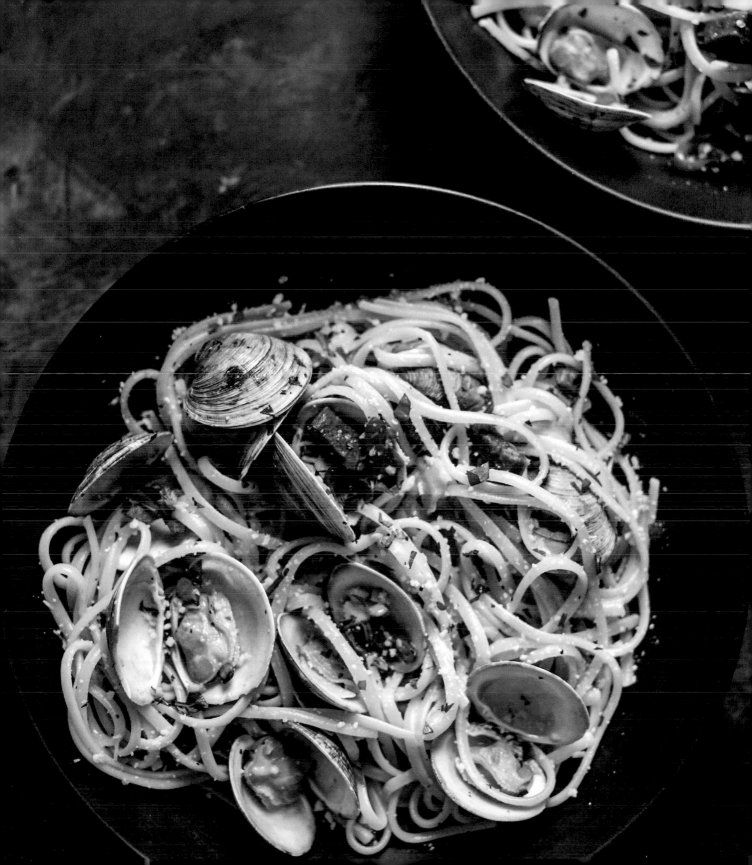

SERVES 2

→ GLUTEN-FREE

→ DAIRY-FREE

→ PALEO IF MODIFIED

→ WHOLE30 IF MODIFIED

→ GRAIN-FREE

Total time: 40 MINUTES

SKILLET CHICKEN *with* WHITE WINE, HERBS, *and* ROASTED BROCCOLINI

1 pound boneless, skinless chicken cutlets

½ teaspoon kosher salt, or more to taste

¼ teaspoon freshly ground black pepper

2 tablespoons arrowroot starch

2 tablespoons extra virgin olive oil

1 tablespoon ghee or butter

¼ cup finely diced shallot (1 large)

2 cloves garlic, very thinly sliced

2 cups thinly sliced baby bella mushrooms (about 6)

1 cup dry white wine (substitute 1 cup chicken broth plus 1 tablespoon fresh lemon juice for Whole30, paleo)

1 teaspoon fresh rosemary leaves (1 sprig)

1 teaspoon fresh thyme leaves (4 sprigs)

2 tablespoons chopped fresh flat-leaf parsley leaves

Easy Oven-Roasted Broccolini (recipe follows)

Cooking with wine is fun. I'm not talking about just holding a glass of wine while cooking (although that's pretty great, too), but actually putting the wine in your dish and cooking with it. Don't worry, it won't make you tipsy or anything as the alcohol in the wine evaporates while the food is cooking. Only the flavor remains. Boiling down the wine concentrates the flavor, including acidity and sweetness—resulting in an absolutely delicious dish. Here, I've taken some simple chicken cutlets and completely elevated them to a lovable date-night dish by cooking them in white wine and lots of lovely herbs. It's simple, yet so sophisticated and one that you'll just adore.

Season both sides of the chicken cutlets with salt and pepper. Place the arrowroot on a separate plate. Individually dredge both sides of the chicken by dipping them into the arrowroot so that they are lightly coated on both sides in the flour. Shake off any excess flour (you don't want it layered on too thick, or it won't crisp up nicely).

Heat a skillet over medium-high heat with olive oil. When the oil is shimmering, swirl the pan so the oil evenly coats the bottom of the skillet. Place the chicken into the skillet and brown on both sides until a nice golden brown crust has formed, about 3 minutes per side. Once browned, remove the chicken to a plate and set aside.

{ continued }

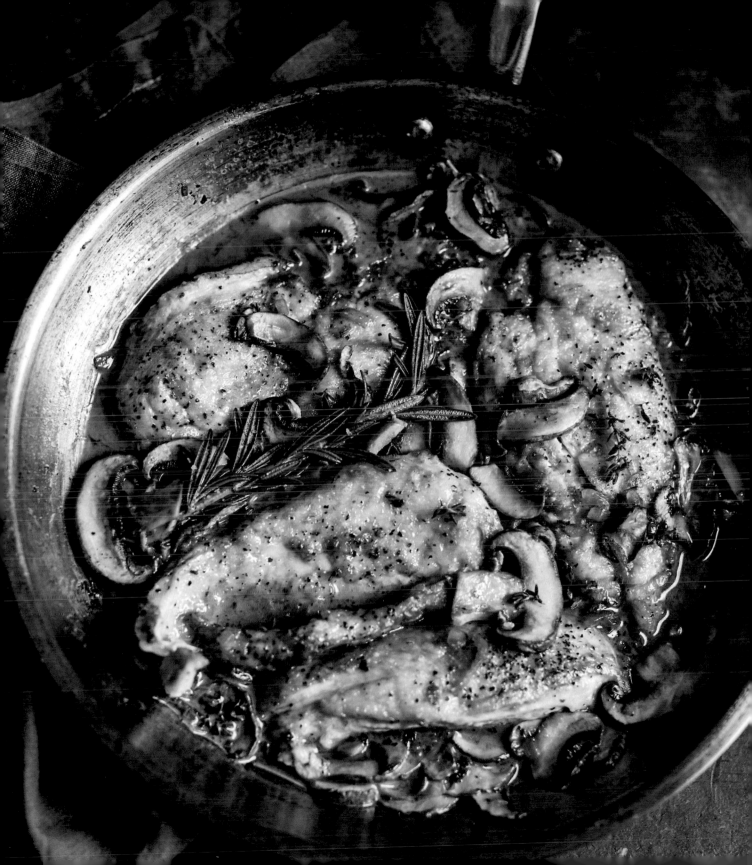

Reduce the heat to medium, add the butter or ghee, and let melt. Add the shallot and cook, stirring, until tender, about 2 minutes. Add the garlic and mushrooms and cook, stirring, for about 2 more minutes to let the mushrooms develop some flavor. Pour in the white wine, rosemary, and thyme and cook, stirring, until the mushrooms are tender, about 2 minutes.

Nestle the browned chicken into the white wine sauce and adjust the heat so that the sauce is simmering. Cook until the sauce has thickened and chicken is cooked through, about 8 more minutes.

Top with fresh parsley and serve with the broccolini.

EASY OVEN-ROASTED BROCCOLINI

TOTAL TIME: 15 minutes

- 1 head broccolini, trimmed
- 1 tablespoon extra virgin olive oil
- ¼ teaspoon crushed red pepper flakes
- ¼ teaspoon kosher salt
- ¼ teaspoon freshly ground black pepper
- 1 tablespoon fresh lemon juice (½ lemon)

Preheat the oven to 400°F and line a baking sheet with parchment paper.

Place the broccolini on the prepared baking sheet and drizzle with the olive oil, red pepper flakes, salt, and pepper. Toss to coat evenly and spread in a single layer across the baking sheet.

Transfer to the oven and bake until tender and the edges are slightly golden-brown and crisp, about 15 minutes. Remove from the oven and drizzle with the lemon juice.

from
MY KITCHEN
to YOURS

This recipe goes great with anything starchy and anything green. I pair mine with oven-roasted broccolini and a side of mashed potatoes. You could also serve it over pasta or steamed rice.

BLUEBERRY FILET MIGNON *with* CAULIFLOWER MASH

SERVES 2
→ GLUTEN-FREE
→ DAIRY-FREE
→ PALEO
→ GRAIN-FREE
Total time: 45 MINUTES

One of my most favorite cities in the world is Florence, Italy. This Renaissance city is oh-so-enchanting, not to mention the best place to feast on world-class art and gourmet cuisine. I will never forget trying the blueberry steak at the local restaurant Acqua al Due. When the waiter recommended we order it for our dinner, I had my hesitation, but decided to trust the expert. And I am so glad that I did! Sweet and savory, this is a dish that begs for a serving and is best enjoyed with your companion for a special night.

MAKE THE SAUCE In a small saucepan, heat the olive oil over medium heat. Add the shallot, garlic, and red pepper flakes and gently cook until tender, about 3 minutes.

Add the blueberries, balsamic vinegar, palm sugar, and rosemary. Bring the sauce to a boil, then reduce the heat to a light simmer. Cook, stirring occasionally, until the sauce has thickened and coats the back of a spoon, about 20 minutes. Taste and add salt if necessary.

Remove the rosemary sprig and discard. You can either keep the sauce as is or, for a smoother sauce, use an immersion blender (or working in batches in a blender), blend the sauce until smooth. Cover the sauce to keep it warm while you prepare the rest of the dish.

MAKE THE MASH In a large pot with a tight-fitting lid, combine the cauliflower florets, broth, and garlic. Cover the pot and bring the broth to a boil over high heat. Let the cauliflower steam until fork tender, about 15 minutes. Do not drain. Add the coconut

{ continued }

FOR THE BLUEBERRY SAUCE

- 2 tablespoons extra virgin olive oil
- 1 medium shallot, very finely diced (¼ cup)
- 1 garlic clove, minced
- ¼ teaspoon crushed red pepper flakes
- 1 pint fresh blueberries
- ¼ cup aged balsamic vinegar
- 1 tablespoon coconut palm sugar
- 1 sprig fresh rosemary
  Kosher salt

FOR THE CAULIFLOWER MASH

- 2 small heads cauliflower, cut into florets (8 cups)
- 2 cups low-sodium chicken broth
- 2 garlic cloves
- ½ cup unsweetened full-fat coconut milk
- 1 teaspoon kosher salt
- ½ teaspoon freshly ground black pepper

FOR THE STEAKS

- 2 (8-ounce) filets mignons, 1 inch thick (see Note)
- 1 teaspoons kosher salt
- ½ teaspoon freshly ground black pepper
- 2 tablespoons avocado oil

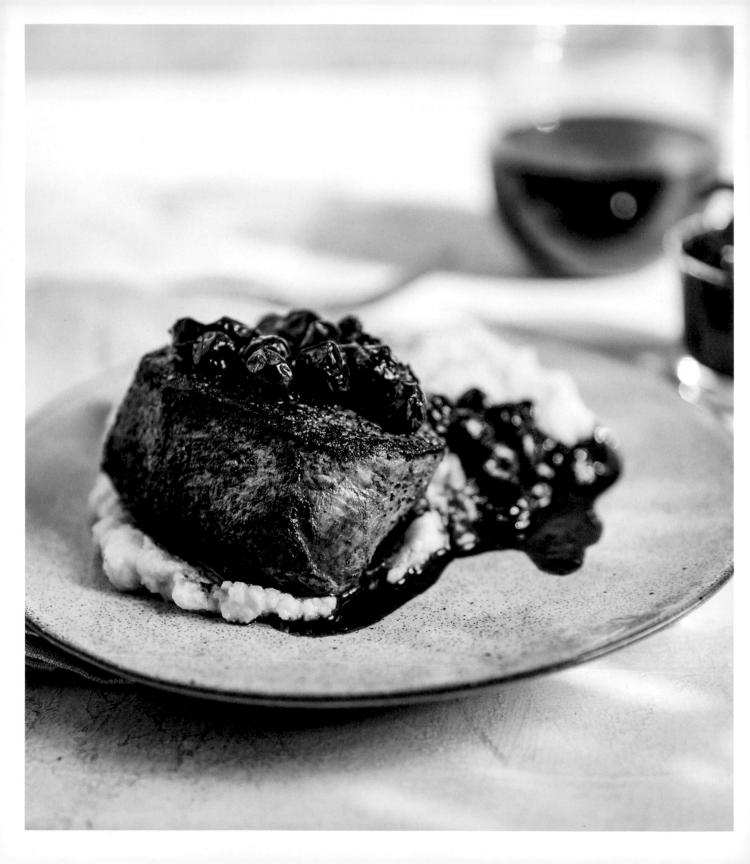

milk, salt, and pepper and using an immersion blender or working in batches in a blender, blend the cauliflower mixture until smooth. Cover and keep warm until ready to serve.

MAKE THE STEAKS Pat the steaks dry with a paper towel, then season both sides of the steak generously with the salt and pepper.

Heat the avocado oil in a large cast-iron skillet over high heat until it just begins to smoke. Use a pair of tongs to carefully place the steaks in the skillet. Cook until a deep brown crust forms on each side, about 4 minutes per side for medium-rare or 5 to 6 minutes per side if you like your steak a little more well done. Transfer the steaks to a cutting board to rest for 10 minutes before serving.

Drizzle the steaks with the sauce and serve alongside the cauliflower mash.

from
MY KITCHEN
to YOURS

When I cook steaks, I always remove them from the fridge and let rest at room temperature for 20 minutes prior to cooking. This way, they aren't cold and don't seize when they hit the pan, resulting in more tender, evenly cooked steaks!

SERVES 2

→ GLUTEN-FREE

→ DAIRY-FREE

→ PALEO IF MODIFIED

→ WHOLE30 IF MODIFIED

→ GRAIN-FREE

Total time: 40 MINUTES

PAN-ROASTED BLACKENED CAJUN CHICKEN *with* OVEN FRITES

1 teaspoon kosher salt

½ teaspoon freshly ground black pepper

½ teaspoon dried thyme

½ teaspoon cayenne pepper

½ teaspoon paprika

¼ teaspoon dried rosemary

¼ teaspoon dried oregano

2 boneless, skin-on chicken breasts (about 1½ pounds) (ask your butcher!)

1 tablespoon avocado oil

½ cup dry white wine (substitute ½ cup low-sodium chicken broth plus 1 teaspoon lemon juice for Whole30, paleo)

½ cup low-sodium chicken broth

½ teaspoon arrowroot starch

1 garlic clove, minced

2 tablespoons unsalted butter or ghee (use ghee for Whole30, paleo)

1 tablespoon fresh lemon juice (½ lemon)

Oven Frites (recipe follows)

After you make this recipe, you're going to feel like you need to open a restaurant. It's the juiciest, most flavorful, professional chef–quality chicken that you could possibly make in your very own kitchen—and using only clean ingredients. Sold yet?!

The inspiration for this dish came from one of Clayton and my favorite Dallas date-night restaurants, Le Bilboquet, where they serve a Cajun spice–rubbed chicken with frites. Without fail, I order it every single time we go. And considering that it's one of my favorite date-night dinners, it seemed only fitting that I include my at-home, cleaned-up version in the date-night chapter of this book. I hope you enjoy and seriously impress your date!

Preheat the oven to 400°F.

In a small bowl, combine the salt, pepper, thyme, cayenne pepper, paprika, rosemary, and oregano. Set aside.

Pat the chicken breasts dry and season the skin side with half of the spice mixture.

In a medium oven-safe skillet, heat the avocado oil over medium-high heat until just starting to smoke. Carefully lay the chicken breasts into the hot skillet skin-side down. Cook without moving until the skin is a deep golden brown and very crisp, about 6 minutes. While cooking, season the second side of the chicken

{ continued }

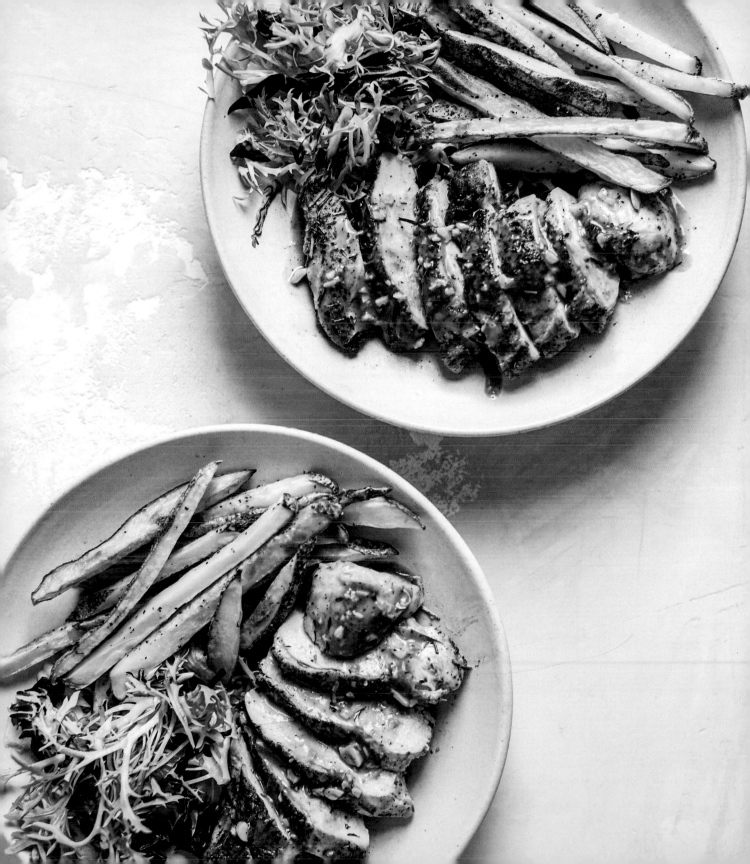

with the remaining spice mixture. Carefully flip the chicken breasts and transfer the skillet to the oven. Bake until cooked through, or when an instant-read thermometer inserted into the thickest part of the breasts registers 150°F, 12 to 15 minutes. Reserving the pan juices in the skillet, transfer the chicken to a cutting board and set aside.

In a medium bowl, combine the wine, chicken broth, and arrowroot and whisk until the arrowroot dissolves. Set aside.

Pour off all but about 1 teaspoon of the fat from the skillet and place the pan over high heat. Add the garlic along with the wine mixture, scraping up any browned bits from the bottom of the skillet. Cook, stirring, until the sauce reduces by two-thirds, about 5 minutes. Remove the pan from the heat and add the butter and the lemon juice and allow the butter to just melt. Stir to combine. Taste the pan sauce and season with more salt and pepper, if desired.

Slice the chicken breasts and serve on individual plates. Spoon plenty of pan sauce over the sliced chicken and serve with the oven frites.

OVEN FRITES

TOTAL TIME: 40 minutes

- 1½ pounds russet potatoes (or 2 large potatoes)
- 2 tablespoons extra virgin olive oil
- 1½ teaspoons kosher salt
- ½ teaspoon freshly ground black pepper

Preheat the oven to 400°F and line a large baking sheet with parchment paper.

Scrub the potatoes well, then cut lengthwise into ½-inch-wide fries.

Place the fries in a large bowl and toss with the olive oil, salt, and pepper until evenly coated.

Spread the fries across the prepared baking sheet in a single layer (you may need two baking sheets to ensure they are in a single layer and have plenty of room to crisp up).

Bake in the oven until the potatoes are golden brown all over and crisp, about 30 minutes (and no, you do not need to toss during the cooking time at all).

WALNUT-CRUSTED SCALLOPS *with* BUTTERNUT SQUASH PUREE

SERVES 2
→ GLUTEN-FREE
→ DAIRY-FREE
→ PALEO
→ WHOLE30
→ GRAIN-FREE
Total time: 30 MINUTES

Table for two, please! At the house! Date night comes in 30 minutes or less with this dish. It's a little bit fancy with a huge amount of flavor, and yet so super-easy to cook up. You and your sweetheart will just love this cozy—and healthy—dish.

MAKE THE PUREE In a medium saucepan, combine the butternut squash, broth, and garlic and turn to medium-high heat. Bring to a boil and cover. Cook until the squash is very tender, 15 to 20 minutes.

Transfer the contents of the saucepan (do not drain) to a high-powered blender or food processor. Add the coconut milk, salt, and thyme and puree in 20-second increments, scraping down the sides after each blending session, and blending until very smooth. Return the puree to the saucepan and cover to keep warm until ready to serve.

MAKE THE SCALLOPS Combine the walnuts, garlic powder and paprika in a large resealable food-storage bag. Seal the bag and use a meat mallet or the back of a skillet to crush the walnuts until they are a similar texture to panko breadcrumbs. Transfer the walnut mixture to a large plate.

Spread the scallops in a single layer on a paper towel and pat dry. Season both sides with the salt and pepper.

{ continued }

FOR THE BUTTERNUT SQUASH PUREE

- 4 cups butternut squash, peeled, seeded and cut into 1-inch cubes (1 large)
- 1 cup low-sodium chicken broth
- 1 garlic clove
- ¼ cup unsweetened full-fat coconut milk
- ½ teaspoon kosher salt
- ¼ teaspoon dried thyme

FOR THE SCALLOPS

- ⅔ cup unsalted walnuts
- ½ teaspoon garlic powder
- ¼ teaspoon smoked paprika
- 1 pound sea scallops
- 1 teaspoon kosher salt
- ½ teaspoon freshly ground black pepper
- 2 tablespoons extra virgin olive oil
- 1 tablespoon finely chopped fresh flat-leaf parsley leaves, for serving

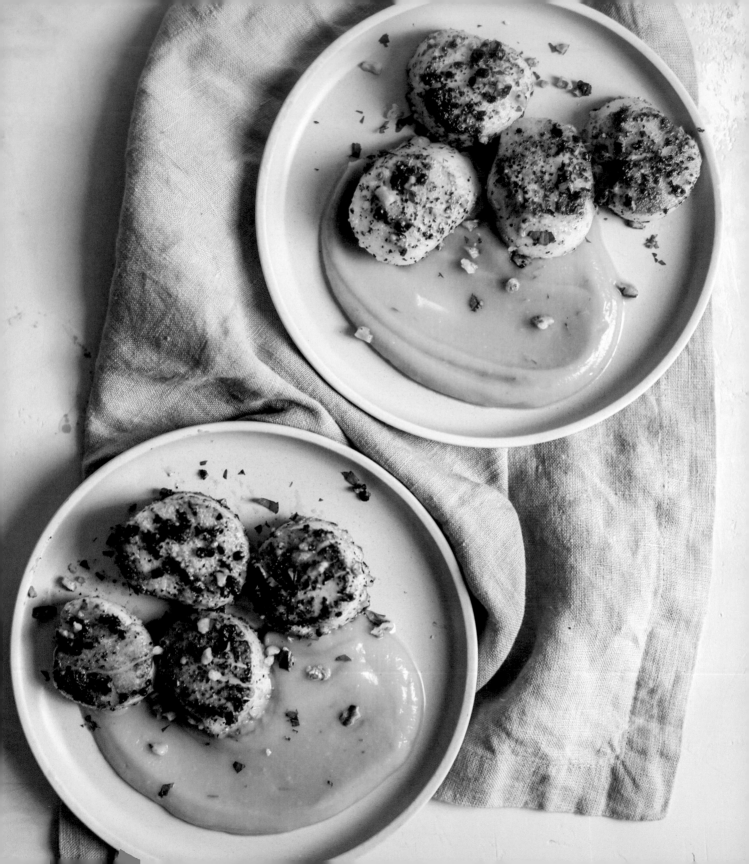

In a large skillet, heat the olive oil over medium-high heat until it shimmers. Swirl the pan so the olive oil evenly coats the bottom. Dip both sides of each scallop into the walnut crumbs to coat each end like a crust. Working in batches so as to not crowd the pan, add the scallops to the skillet. Cook until the scallops are golden brown on each side and cooked through, about 2 minutes per side. Transfer the cooked scallops to a paper-lined plate and repeat with the remaining scallops.

To serve, divide the butternut squash puree between 2 serving bowls and top with the scallops. Sprinkle with parsley.

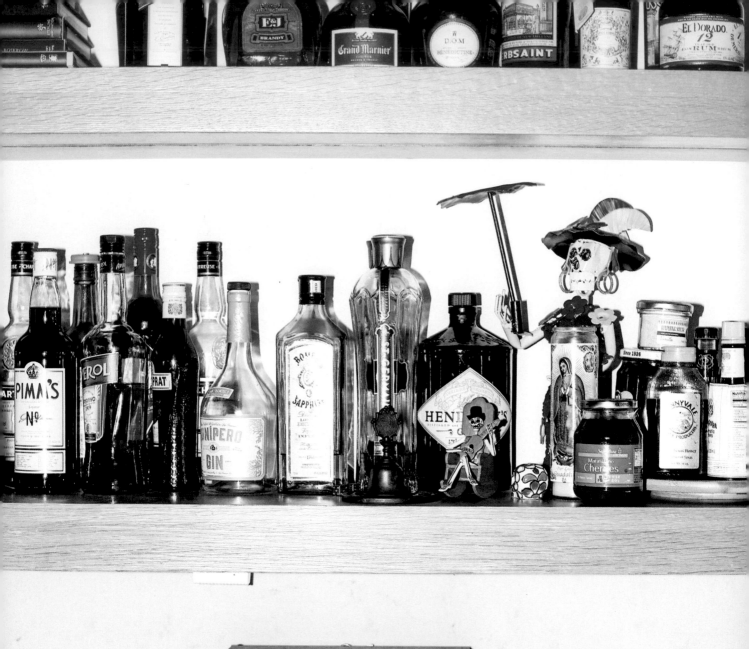

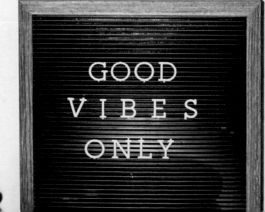

GOOD
VIBES
ONLY

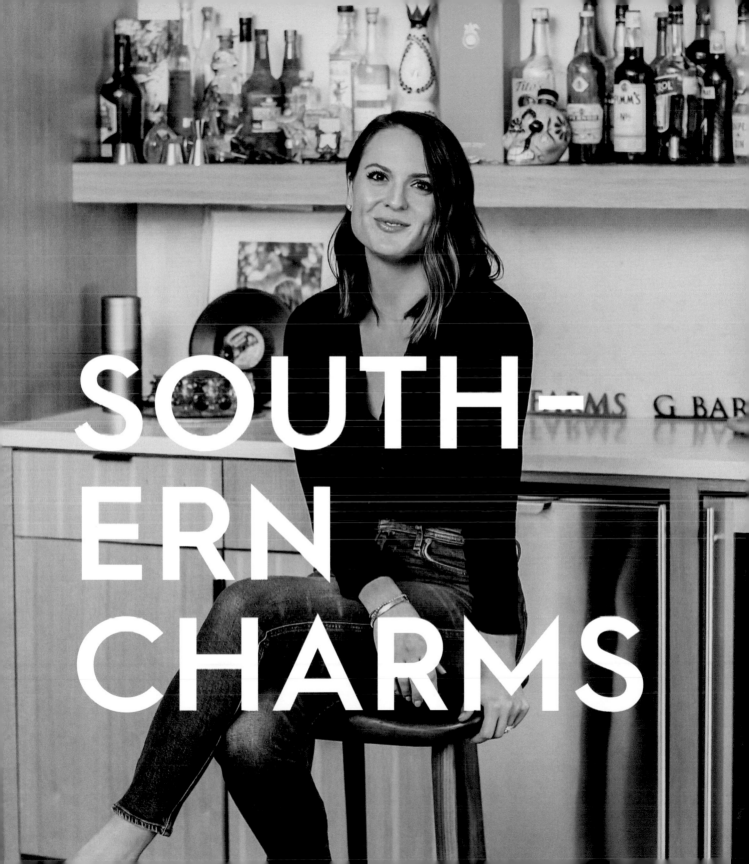

SOUTHERN CHARMS

SERVES 4

→ GLUTEN-FREE

→ DAIRY-FREE

→ PALEO

→ WHOLE30

→ GRAIN-FREE

Total time: 40 MINUTES

NASHVILLE UN-FRIED HOT CHICKEN *with* EASY COLLARD GREENS

2 pounds bone-in, skin-on chicken thighs

1 teaspoon kosher salt

½ teaspoon freshly ground black pepper

2 tablespoons avocado oil

2 tablespoons ghee

2 tablespoons Tabasco sauce

1 teaspoon white vinegar

1 teaspoon coconut aminos

2 garlic cloves, minced

½ teaspoon cayenne pepper

½ teaspoon chili powder

½ teaspoon smoked paprika

Easy Collard Greens (recipe follows)

Nothing says the South like some good ole deep-fried chicken. Bonus points if it's smothered in a hot and spicy sauce. That's what you get with Nashville Hot Chicken, aka pure southern bliss. As a girl who loves spicy and loves crispy chicken, this dish speaks to my soul. But I am certainly not going to be deep-frying chicken on a weeknight—it's not what I'm about health- or time-wise. There's of course a time and place to splurge on fried chicken, but a Wednesday night in my kitchen just isn't one of them! So, I've taken bone-in skin-on chicken thighs, pan-roasted them until they are as crispy as they can possibly get, and tossed them in a fabulous hot sauce for a cleaned-up "un-fried" chicken that will knock your socks off. Paired with some Easy Collard Greens (recipe follows), you have one heck of a Southern comfort weeknight meal.

Preheat the oven to 475°F.

Pat the chicken thighs dry and generously season all over with the salt and pepper.

Heat the avocado oil in a large oven-safe skillet, preferably cast-iron, over medium-high heat until very hot but not smoking. Add the chicken skin-side down and sear, occasionally rearranging the chicken thighs and rotating the pan to evenly distribute the heat, until the fat renders and the skin is golden brown, 7 to 8 minutes. Leave in their skin-side

{ continued }

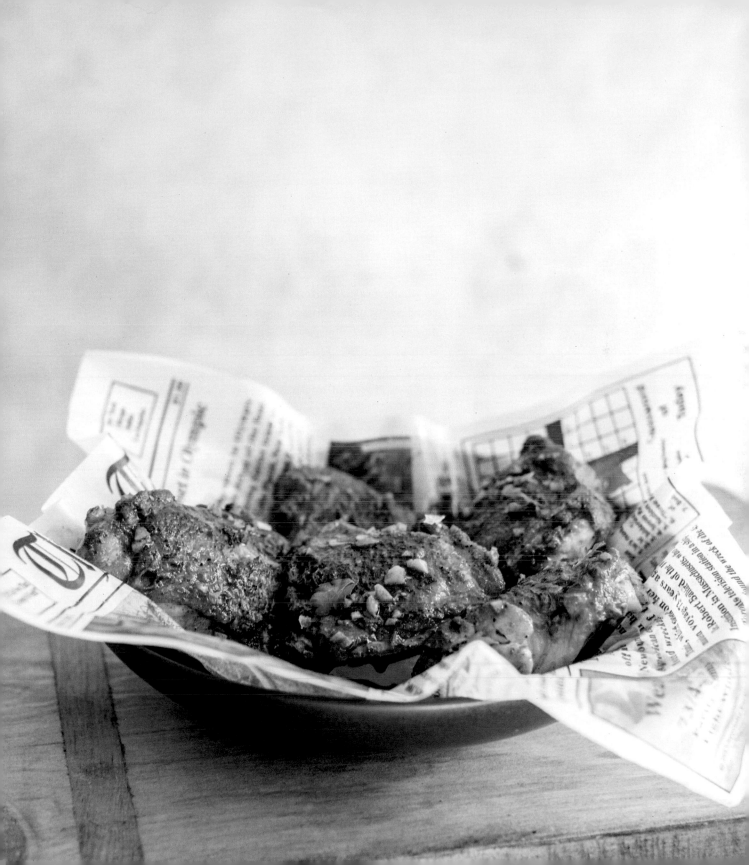

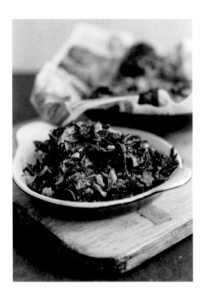

TOTAL TIME: 30 minutes

2 bunches collard greens, rinsed

4 strips sugar- and nitrate-free bacon, diced into ½-inch pieces (I use Pederson's Natural Farms brand)

½ medium yellow onion, finely diced (1 cup)

3 garlic cloves, minced

½ teaspoon crushed red pepper flakes

½ cup low-sodium chicken broth

2 tablespoons apple cider vinegar

Kosher salt and freshly ground black pepper

down position and transfer the skillet to the oven. Roast for 10 more minutes.

Carefully flip the chicken skin-side up and continue roasting until the meat is cooked through, about 3 minutes longer. Transfer the chicken to a large bowl and let it rest 5 to 10 minutes before serving.

Meanwhile, heat a small saucepan over medium heat and combine the ghee, Tabasco, vinegar, coconut aminos, garlic, cayenne pepper, chili powder, and paprika. Bring the sauce to a simmer and cook, uncovered and whisking often, until the sauce is fragrant and the flavors have combined, 3 to 5 minutes.

Pour the sauce over the chicken and toss to coat well. Serve immediately with Easy Collard Greens.

EASY COLLARD GREENS

Strip the leaves from the tough stems of the collard greens and discard the stems. Stack the leaves on a cutting board and roll them up, like a cigar, and slice into thin strips. Set aside.

Heat a large high-sided skillet or pot over medium heat. Add the diced bacon and cook, stirring occasionally, until browned, about 5 minutes. Add the onion and cook until tender, about 3 minutes. Stir in the garlic and red pepper flakes and gently cook, stirring and being careful not to burn the garlic, for 1 minute.

Pour in the chicken broth and use your spoon to scrape up the browned bits from the bottom of the pan. Add the shredded collard greens and the apple cider vinegar and cook, stirring, until the collards have wilted down a bit and are completely submerged in the broth mixture, about 3 minutes. Reduce the heat to medium-low, cover, and cook, stirring occasionally, until the collards are tender and no longer bitter, 15 to 20 minutes. Season with salt and pepper to taste.

CAJUN CRAB CAKES *with* REMOULADE

SERVES 4
→ GLUTEN-FREE
→ DAIRY-FREE
→ PALEO
→ WHOLE30
→ GRAIN-FREE

Total time: 45 MINUTES

You've probably figured out by now that I'm partial to big, bold, spicy flavors. This, in turn, makes me one of the biggest fans of Cajun food of all time. So I knew just where to start looking in terms of inspiration when it came time to make over my classic crab cake recipe. My classic crab cakes are one of the most popular on my site thanks to the lovely actress and film producer, Emmy Rossum, making them and posting about it on her social media account. Here, I've jazzed them up with a dash of zesty flavor from bell peppers and cayenne pepper, plus a creamy remoulade dipping sauce make these new-and-improved crab cakes 100-percent Cajun-approved. You'd never guess that they're Whole30 and paleo-compliant!

MAKE THE REMOULADE In a medium bowl, combine the mayo, mustard, lemon juice, parsley, green onion, garlic, capers, hot sauce, relish, apple cider vinegar, paprika, salt, and cayenne pepper. Stir to combine. Cover and refrigerate until ready to serve.

MAKE THE CRAB CAKES Line a large baking sheet with parchment paper and set aside.

In a large bowl, combine the crabmeat, bell pepper, green onions, mayo, cassava flour, salt, red pepper flakes, black pepper, cayenne pepper, and thyme. Use a fork to mix until just combined.

Use a ½-cup measuring cup to scoop out the crab mixture and, using your hands, form into patties. Set on the prepared baking sheet and refrigerate for about 20 minutes to allow them

{ continued }

FOR THE REMOULADE

- ½ cup homemade mayo (page 281)
- 1 tablespoon creole or Dijon mustard
- 1 tablespoon fresh lemon juice (½ lemon)
- 1 tablespoon finely chopped fresh flat-leaf parsley leaves
- 1 green onion (white and green parts), finely chopped
- 2 garlic cloves, minced
- 1 teaspoon capers, roughly chopped
- 1 teaspoon Louisiana-style hot sauce (I use Crystal brand)
- 1 teaspoon dill relish, no sugar added
- ½ teaspoon apple cider vinegar
- ½ teaspoon paprika
- ½ teaspoon kosher salt
- ⅛ teaspoon cayenne pepper

FOR THE CRAB CAKES
(on following page)

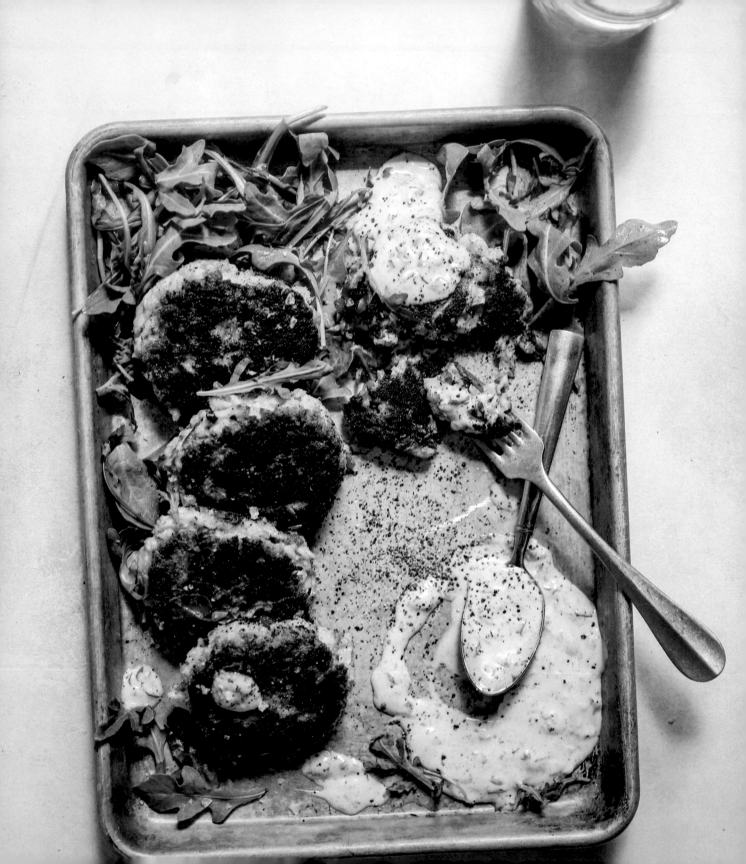

FOR THE CRAB CAKES

16 ounces fresh lump crabmeat (if you buy canned, be sure to drain it first)

½ red bell pepper, seeded and finely diced (½ cup)

2 green onions (white and green parts), thinly sliced (½ cup)

¼ cup plus 1 teaspoon homemade mayo (page 281)

1 tablespoon plus 1 teaspoon cassava flour

1 teaspoon kosher salt

½ teaspoon crushed red pepper flakes

¼ teaspoon freshly ground black pepper

¼ teaspoon cayenne pepper

¼ teaspoon dried thyme

¼ cup almond flour

2 tablespoons extra virgin olive oil

to firm up. This helps prevent the patties from falling apart when coating them with almond flour and cooking them.

Pour the almond flour onto a plate. Very lightly dredge each chilled crab cake in the flour and tap off any excess flour. You don't want them caked in flour or they'll taste dry, just lightly dusted. Return the coated crab cakes to the baking sheet.

In a large nonstick skillet, heat the olive oil over medium-high heat. When the oil is very hot but not smoking, carefully arrange the crab cakes in the bottom of the skillet, taking care not to crowd the pan. You will most likely have to do this in batches. Sear the patties until they are golden brown and slightly crispy, 3 to 4 minutes on the first side. Use a sturdy spatula to carefully flip the patties and cook for 3 more minutes on the second side. Transfer cooked crab cakes to a wire rack to keep them from getting soggy before serving. Repeat with the remaining crab cakes.

Serve hot with the remoulade and enjoy.

SERVES 4

→ GLUTEN-FREE

→ DAIRY-FREE

→ PALEO

→ WHOLE30

→ GRAIN-FREE

Total time: 35 MINUTES

CHICKEN-FRIED STEAK *with* CREAMY CAULIFLOWER GRAVY

FOR THE CREAMY CAULIFLOWER GRAVY

- 2 tablespoons ghee
- 1 cup diced yellow onion (1 medium)
- 1 teaspoon kosher salt
- ½ teaspoon dried thyme
- 4 cups fresh cauliflower florets (1 large head)
- 2 cups low-sodium chicken broth
- 1 teaspoon freshly ground black pepper

FOR THE CHICKEN-FRIED STEAK

- ½ cup almond flour
- ½ cup tapioca starch
- 3 teaspoons kosher salt
- 1 teaspoon garlic powder
- 1 teaspoon onion powder
- 1 teaspoon smoked paprika
- 1 teaspoon freshly ground black pepper, plus more for serving
- ½ teaspoon cayenne pepper
- 3 large eggs
- ½ cup avocado oil
- 4 (6-ounce) beef cube steaks
  Dried thyme, for serving

Whoever invented chicken-fried steak is an evil genius. If you aren't familiar with this Southern favorite, it's tenderized beef cutlets that have been dipped in egg and flour and fried, much like fried chicken, just with steak. Oh, and then they're smothered in gravy. It's pretty much a gut bomb of gluttonous deliciousness, but good grief, is it fantastic!

Well, let's just say that I gave the Southern favorite a Whole30 makeover, and I still can't believe how dang good it is. This grain-free, super-duper crispy fried steak is smothered with a creamy cauliflower gravy. The only way to believe how delicious *and* healthy this is to make it for yourself!

MAKE THE GRAVY In a large saucepan over medium heat, melt the ghee. Add the onion, salt, and thyme and cook until the onion is tender, 3 to 4 minutes.

Add the cauliflower florets and broth and bring to a boil. Reduce the heat to a simmer and let the gravy cook, covered, until the cauliflower is fork-tender, about 15 minutes. Transfer the mixture to a high-powered blender and blend until very smooth. Stir in the black pepper. Cover and keep warm until ready to use.

MAKE THE STEAKS In a bowl, combine the almond flour, tapioca starch, 2 teaspoons of the salt, garlic powder, onion powder,

{ continued }

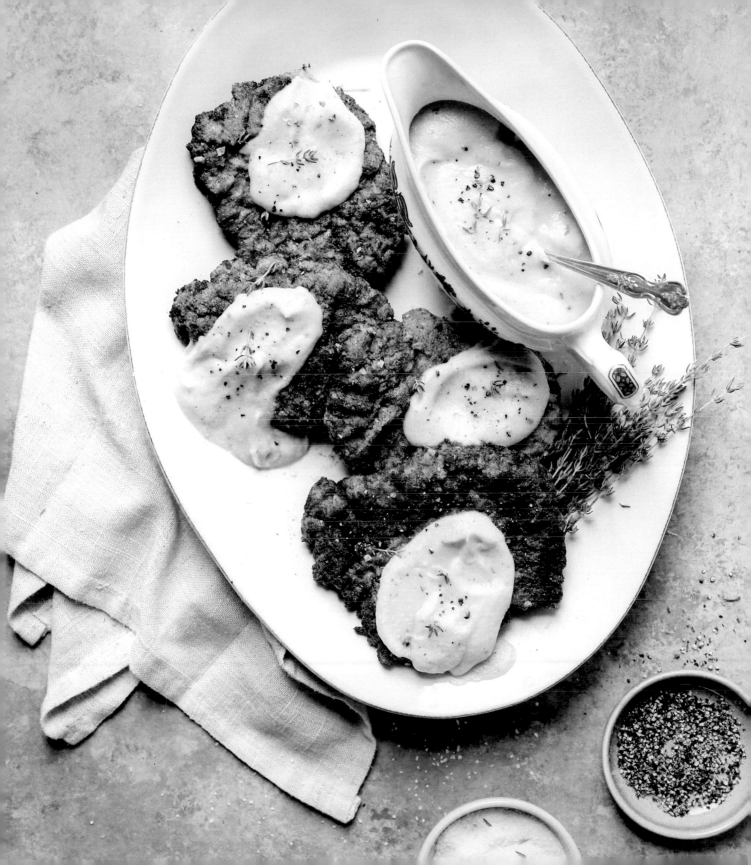

paprika, ½ teaspoon of black pepper, and cayenne pepper. Using a fork, stir to combine and break up any clumps.

In a separate shallow bowl, combine the eggs and whisk until well combined.

Pat the steaks dry then sprinkle on both sides with the remaining 1 teaspoon salt and ½ teaspoon black pepper.

In a large Dutch oven, heat the avocado oil over medium-high heat.

Just before frying the individual steaks, dip them in the egg wash, then dredge them through the flour mixture to evenly coat. Shake off excess.

Working in batches, fry each steak in the oil until golden brown, crispy, and cooked through, 3 to 4 minutes per side. Use a sturdy spatula to transfer the fried steaks to a wire rack to cool.

To serve, smother the steaks with the gravy and garnish with a sprinkle of thyme and a couple cracks of black pepper.

MEATLOAF MEATBALLS *with* MASHED POTATOES *and* GREEN BEANS

SERVES 4
→ GLUTEN-FREE
→ DAIRY-FREE
→ PALEO
→ WHOLE30
→ GRAIN-FREE
Total time: 45 MINUTES

When I look back on my childhood, meatloaf was one of those things that I hated so very much. As my blog began to grow, my readers begged for a delicious Whole30-friendly meatloaf. I worked and worked on a recipe until finally, I came up with one that has not only become a huge hit, but has also converted me into a meatloaf lover. It's full of rich, deep flavor thanks to tomato paste and dried thyme, and the best part? I've transformed it from a heavy loaf into bite-size meatballs, served up with creamy mashed potatoes and lemony green beans for a fantastic weeknight meal that's guaranteed to be gobbled up.

MAKE THE MEATBALLS Preheat the oven to 350°F. Spray a 12-cup muffin tin with nonstick cooking spray and set aside.

In a large skillet, heat the ghee over medium heat. Add the onion and thyme and cook, stirring occasionally, until the onion is tender, about 5 minutes. Stir in the tomato paste and coconut aminos and remove the pan from the heat. Set aside to cool.

In a large bowl, combine the ground beef, almond flour, egg, salt, and pepper with the cooled onion mixture. Use a fork to mix until just combined. Use your hands to roll the meat mixture into 12 large meatballs (about 2 tablespoons each). Place an individual meatball in each muffin cup. Set aside.

{ continued }

FOR THE MEATLOAF MEATBALLS

- 1 teaspoon ghee
- ⅔ cup finely diced yellow onion (⅔ medium)
- 1 teaspoon dried thyme
- 1 tablespoon tomato paste
- 1 tablespoon coconut aminos
- 1½ pounds ground beef (80 percent lean)
- ¼ cup almond flour
- 1 large egg, beaten
- 1 teaspoon kosher salt
- ½ teaspoon freshly ground black pepper

FOR THE SAUCE

- 2 tablespoons coconut aminos
- 1 tablespoon tomato paste
- 2 teaspoons Louisiana-style hot sauce (I like Crystal brand)
- 1 teaspoon yellow mustard
- 1 teaspoon garlic powder

Whole30 Mashed Potatoes (recipe follows)

Lemon-Garlic Green Beans (recipe follows)

MAKE THE SAUCE In a small bowl, stir together the coconut aminos, tomato paste, hot sauce, mustard, and garlic powder. Spoon 1 teaspoon of the sauce over each meatball and use the back of the spoon, or a pastry brush, to evenly coat the top.

Bake the meatballs for 25 to 30 minutes, or until the meat is cooked through, or no longer pink, when you cut into a meatball. Let the meatballs cool for 10 minutes before serving. Serve with the Whole30 Mashed Potatoes and Lemon-Garlic Green Beans.

WHOLE30 MASHED POTATOES

TOTAL TIME: 25 minutes

- 2 pounds large yellow potatoes, peeled and cut into 2-inch cubes
- 2 tablespoons ghee
- 2 garlic cloves, minced
- 1 cup low-sodium chicken broth
- ¼ cup unsweetened full-fat coconut milk
- 1 teaspoon kosher salt
- ½ teaspoon freshly ground black pepper

Place the potatoes in a large saucepan and add enough water to cover them by 1 inch. Bring the pot to a boil and cook, covered, until the potatoes are fork-tender, about 15 minutes. Drain the water from the potatoes and set them aside to cool.

While the potatoes are cooling, in the same saucepan, heat the ghee over medium heat. Add the garlic and cook, stirring and being careful not to burn, until the garlic is fragrant, about 2 minutes. Return the potatoes to the pot and add the broth, coconut milk, salt, and pepper and stir to combine. Using a potato masher, mash until the potatoes are smooth and creamy. Keep over medium heat until the potatoes are just reheated through, 3 to 5 more minutes. Taste and adjust the seasoning with more salt and pepper, if desired.

{ continued }

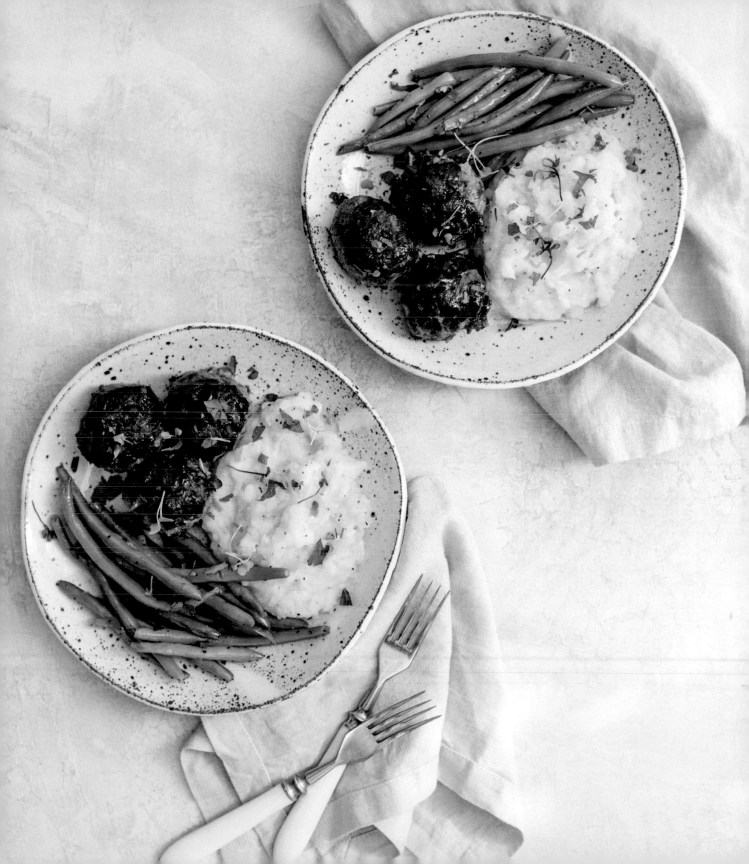

LEMON-GARLIC GREEN BEANS

TOTAL TIME: 15 minutes

12 ounces fresh green beans

1 tablespoon extra virgin olive oil

1 tablespoon fresh lemon juice (½ lemon)

½ teaspoon kosher salt

¼ teaspoon freshly ground black pepper

Fill a large saucepan three-fourths full with water and bring to a boil. Add the green beans and cook until bright green and just beginning to soften, about 3 minutes. Drain the green beans and blanch them by running cold water over them to stop the cooking process. Shake off any excess water and set aside.

Heat the olive oil in a large skillet over medium-high heat. Add the green beans, lemon juice, salt, and pepper. Cook until the green beans are slightly blistered and tender, 4 to 5 minutes.

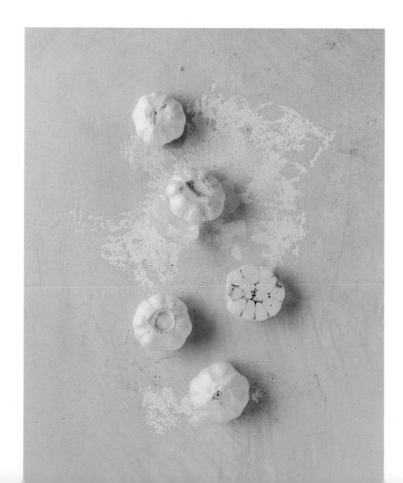

CHICKEN SPAGHETTI SQUASH BOATS

SERVES 4

→ GLUTEN-FREE

→ GRAIN-FREE

Total time: 1 HOUR 15 MINUTES

Growing up in small town Texas, I learned a lot about casseroles. One of the most famous in little ole Celina was Chicken Spaghetti Casserole. Have you ever heard of it? Well, let me just tell you it's comfort food at its finest! In a nut shell, it's spaghetti, chicken, canned soups, and a lot of cheese packed into a casserole dish and baked until bubbly and delicious. It's certainly one of the most epic Southern potluck dishes that people flock to. Here, I've reinvented this Southern classic and made it low-carb by using spaghetti squash. It does have some dairy in it but I can absolutely assure you it's *much better for you* than the casseroles I grew up on. It's filling, full of flavor, easy to make, and oh-so-delicious!

MAKE THE SQUASH Preheat the oven to 400°F and line a large rimmed baking sheet with parchment paper.

Carefully halve spaghetti squash lengthwise by inserting the very tip of a very sharp large knife into the side of the squash (lengthwise) and push it all the way through to the other side. Then rock the knife back and forth to cut one half all the way through, then repeat on the other side until the squash is cut in half.

Scoop and scrape out the seeds and most of the stringy parts of the center of the squash. (I find it's easier if you use an ice cream scoop.)

Brush the interior of the squash with the olive oil and sprinkle with the salt. Place the squash, cut-side down, on the parchment paper–lined baking sheet and roast for 45 minutes, or until a knife easily pierces the skin and flesh. Remove from the oven and set

{ continued }

FOR THE SPAGHETTI SQUASH

- 2 medium-sized spaghetti squash
- 2 tablespoons extra virgin olive oil
- ½ teaspoon kosher salt

FOR THE BOATS

- 1 (4-ounce) jar diced pimientos, drained
- 1 (4-ounce) can mild, diced green chiles, drained
- 2 cups small-dice chicken (rotisserie or see page 279)
- ¾ cup small-dice baby bella mushrooms (about 4 mushrooms)
- ¾ cup thinly sliced green onions (white and green parts, 3 to 4), reserve ¼ cup for garnish
- 1 (8-ounce) container sour cream
- 1 teaspoon garlic powder
- 1 teaspoon paprika
- 1½ teaspoons kosher salt
- ½ teaspoon freshly ground black pepper
- 1½ cups shredded sharp cheddar

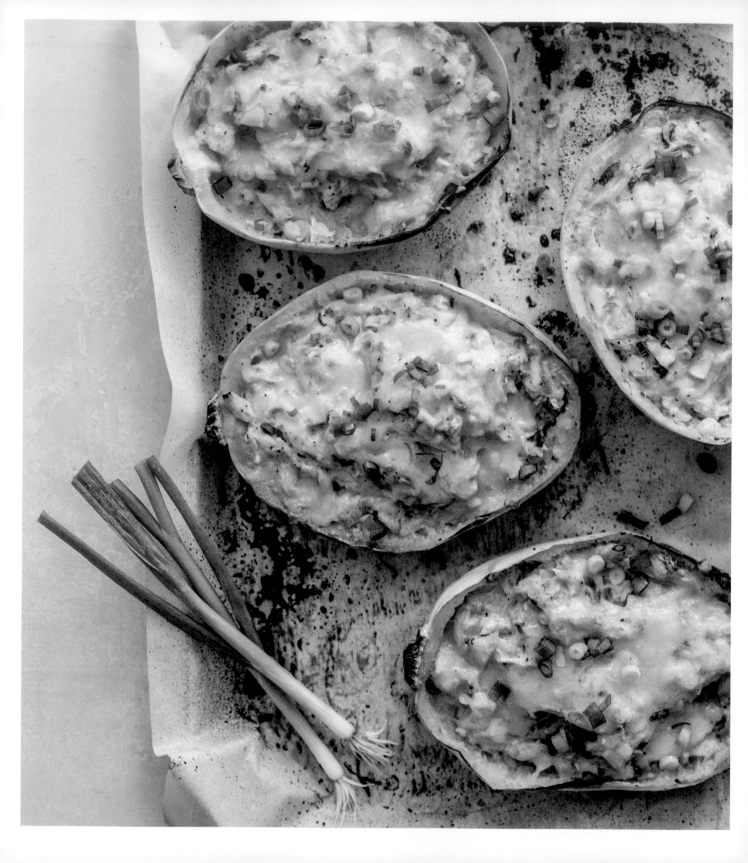

aside until cool enough to handle. (Keep the oven on at this time as they will go back in the oven to finish baking.)

MAKE THE BOATS Meanwhile, in a large bowl, combine the pimientos, green chiles, chicken, mushrooms, ½ cup of the green onions, sour cream, garlic powder, paprika, salt, black pepper, and 1 cup sharp cheddar. When the boats are cool enough to handle, gently scoop out the squash from the shell using a fork to scrape out the strings, being careful not to break the shell. You do not need to get every little bit of squash out of the shell, just get as much as you can as you'll use the shells as boats to serve. Add the spaghetti squash strings to the chicken mixture and toss until well combined.

Place the squash cut-side up on the baking sheet. Divide the mixture evenly among the four squash boats, using the boats as bowls. Sprinkle the remaining ½ cup cheddar on the tops of the boats. Return stuffed boats to the oven and bake for 15 minutes, or until they are hot all the way through and the cheese is melted and bubbly on the top.

Remove from oven and let cool for 5 minutes. Garnish with the remaining green onions.

SERVES 4

→ GLUTEN-FREE

→ DAIRY-FREE

→ PALEO

→ WHOLE30

→ GRAIN-FREE

Total time: 45 MINUTES

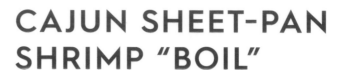

CAJUN SHEET-PAN SHRIMP "BOIL"

1 pound baby red or yellow potatoes, quartered

1 cup diced red bell pepper (1 medium)

12 ounces andouille sausage, fully cooked, sliced into ¼-inch rounds

2 tablespoons extra virgin olive oil

2 teaspoons Old Bay–type seasoning, or more to taste (see Note; I use Primal Palate New Bae)

¾ pound shrimp, peeled and deveined

1 lemon, sliced into ¼-inch rounds

2 tablespoons chopped fresh flat-leaf parsley leaves, for serving

Growing up in the South, attending multiple crawfish boils a year is the norm. Words can't describe the joy of spending a beautiful afternoon with friends and family hovering over a table and eating pounds of crawfish. It's just one of the most wonderful times to share with those you love. Although the real joy is in the social gathering, I also truly enjoy the flavor of a good boil—which is why I've simplified it and made a regular weeknight version that is *so stupid easy.* Literally, just throw all the ingredients on a sheet pan, stick it in the oven, and call it a day! I obviously opted for shrimp instead of crawfish, but the flavors are all there to spice up your weeknight and get dinner on the table in no time.

Preheat the oven to 400°F.

On a parchment-lined baking sheet, combine the potatoes, bell pepper, and sausage. Drizzle with olive oil and season with 1½ teaspoons seasoning. Toss to coat.

Place baking sheet in oven and cook for 20 to 25 minutes, or until the potatoes are tender.

Remove from oven (but keep the oven on) and add the shrimp, lemon slices, and remaining ½ teaspoon seasoning and gently toss to coat evenly with the other ingredients. Return to the oven and cook for an additional 7 to 10 minutes, or until the shrimp is cooked through and pink.

Remove from the oven and gently toss all of the ingredients on the sheet pan to coat in the seasoning. Garnish with the chopped parsley, serve, and enjoy!

from
MY KITCHEN
to YOURS

Most Old Bay–type seasonings are already salted. Check and be sure that yours is. If not, you'll need to season the ingredients with plenty of salt on your own.

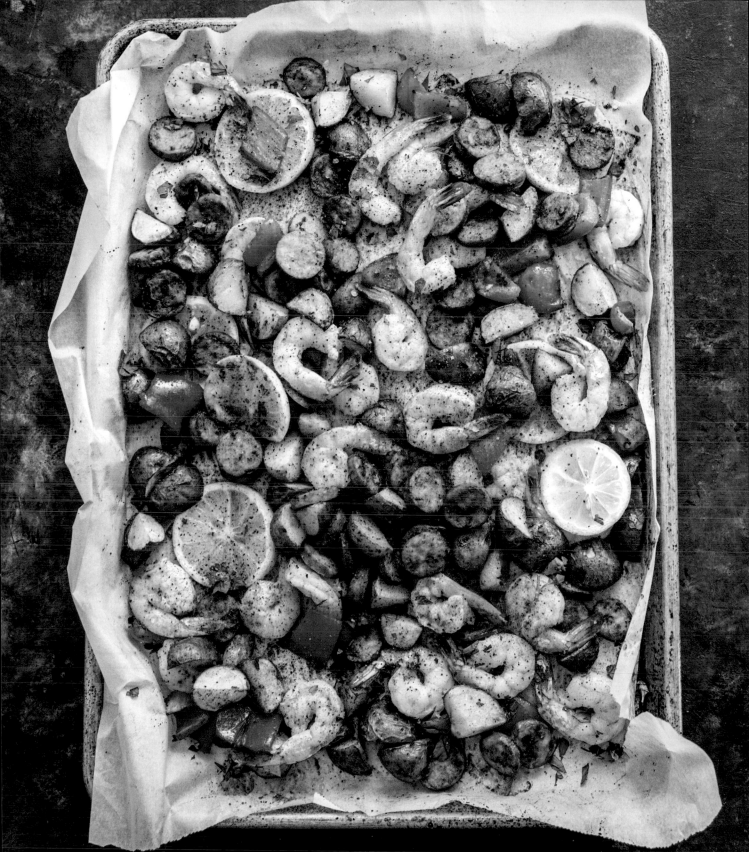

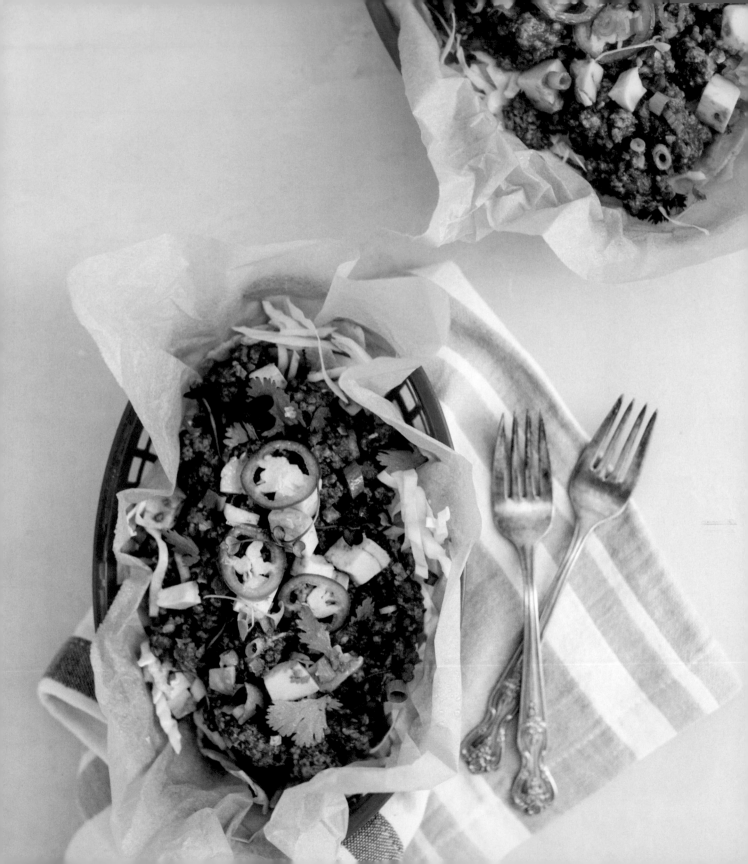

PALEO CHILI PIE

SERVES 6

→ GLUTEN-FREE
→ DAIRY-FREE
→ PALEO
→ GRAIN-FREE

Total time: 40 MINUTES

Please tell me you've had a Frito Chili Pie before. No? Well, I've had about 800 of them in my lifetime—they are a Texas staple—so plenty for the both of us! It's pretty much a football stadium must-have and is essentially corn chips that have been smothered in chili and gooey nacho cheese. What I realized is that you can give this indulgent dish a healthier spin, making it perfect for dinner with your family. I replaced the Fritos with crispy plantain chips and crunchy cabbage, and to make this paleo-friendly, I omitted the beans and cheese. What you're left with is a super flavorful chili spooned over crunchy, crispy bites, and all with the same delicious flavors of the original version.

MAKE THE CHILI In a large skillet, heat the oil over medium heat. Add the onion, jalapeño, and garlic and cook, stirring, until the onion is tender, about 5 minutes.

Increase the heat to medium-high and add the beef, pork, salt, and black pepper. Break up the meat with the back of a spoon and cook until the meat is cooked through and browned, about 7 minutes. Drain off any excess fat.

Add the tomato paste to the browned beef. Stir until well combined. Add the tomato sauce, chili powder, cumin, paprika, apple cider vinegar, and cayenne pepper, if using, plus ¼ cup water. Bring the mixture to a boil, then reduce to a simmer. Continue cooking, uncovered and stirring occasionally, until the flavors have really combined, about 15 minutes. Season with more salt and pepper, if desired.

TO ASSEMBLE Spread about ½ cup of plantain chips over the bottom of 6 serving bowls. Divide the shredded cabbage over each of the bowls. Ladle the chili over the plantains and cabbage and top with avocado, green onion, jalapeño, and cilantro.

FOR THE EASY SKILLET CHILI

- 1 tablespoon avocado oil
- ½ medium yellow onion, finely diced (1 cup)
- 2 tablespoons seeded, finely diced jalapeño (1 medium jalapeño)
- 2 garlic cloves, minced
- 1 pound ground beef, 80 percent lean
- ½ pound ground pork
- 1 teaspoon kosher salt
- ½ teaspoon freshly ground black pepper
- 2 tablespoons tomato paste
- 1 (15-ounce) can tomato sauce
- 1 tablespoon chili powder
- ½ teaspoon ground cumin
- ½ teaspoon sweet paprika
- ½ teaspoon apple cider vinegar
- ¼ teaspoon cayenne pepper (optional)

TO ASSEMBLE

- 3 cups store-bought plain plantain chips (about 2 bags)
- 4 cups finely shredded green cabbage (about ¼ head cabbage)
- 1 avocado, diced
- 2 green onions (green parts only), thinly sliced
- ½ jalapeño, thinly sliced
- 2 tablespoons freshly chopped cilantro leaves

SERVES 4

→ GLUTEN-FREE

→ DAIRY-FREE, IF MODIFIED

Total time: 30 MINUTES

ONE-POT CHICKEN POT PIE PASTA

2 tablespoons extra virgin olive oil

1½ cups small-dice yellow onion (1 large)

1 cup medium-dice carrot (1 large)

1 cup medium-dice celery (2 stalks)

1 teaspoon kosher salt, or more to taste

½ teaspoon freshly ground black pepper, or more to taste

¼ teaspoon cayenne (optional)

12 ounces gluten-free farfalle (or bow tie) pasta (I use Jovial brand brown rice pasta)

2 cups low-sodium chicken broth

2 cups 2 percent milk (for dairy free option, see From My Kitchen To Yours

1 teaspoon dried thyme

1 teaspoon paprika

½ teaspoon dried ground sage

1 teaspoon garlic powder

1 cup frozen peas

2 cups diced chicken (rotisserie or see page 279)

2 tablespoons finely chopped fresh flat-leaf parsley leaves

1 tablespoon lemon juice (or ½ lemon)

Chicken pot pie is one of the most delicious things on earth, it really just is. All of the veggies, the brothy gravy, and the chicken baked underneath a pie crust . . . yum! But, for a weeknight meal it's a pretty big ordeal and a meal with a lot of moving parts. So, here we are taking all of the flavors of the classic chicken pot pie, throwing them in one pot, and making one heck of a weeknight meal. It seriously couldn't be easier and it definitely still has that good-ole comfort food feel. My family just loves this one!

In a Dutch oven or pot, heat the oil over medium heat. When hot, add the onion, carrot, celery, salt, pepper, and cayenne. Cook, stirring, until the veggies are tender, about 6 minutes.

Add in the pasta, chicken broth, milk, thyme, paprika garlic powder, and sage and stir to combine. Bring to a boil. Once boiling, reduce the heat to a simmer and cook, uncovered, stirring occasionally, until the pasta is tender and cooked through, about 12 minutes.

Stir in the frozen peas, diced chicken, parsley, and lemon remove from the heat, and cover. Let it stand until the peas are just cooked through, about 5 more minutes. Taste and add additional seasoning, if desired. Also, if you want your sauce a little thinner, add ¼ cup chicken broth to thin it out.

from
MY KITCHEN
to YOURS

For a dairy-free option, substitute the 2 cups of milk for 1 cup of unsweetened, full-fat coconut milk and 1 cup of water.

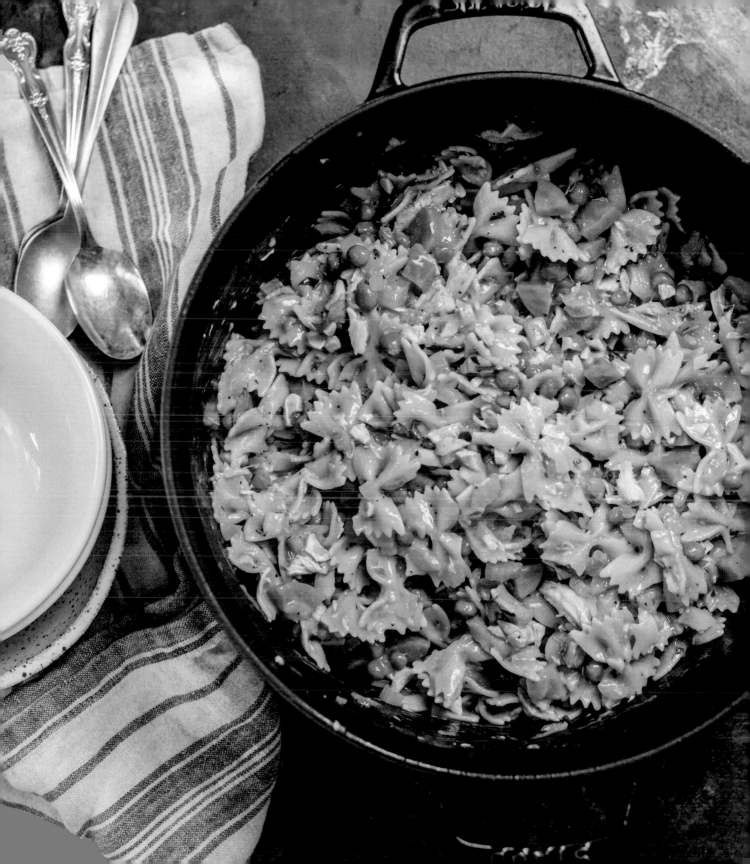

SERVES 4

→ GLUTEN-FREE

→ DAIRY-FREE

→ PALEO

→ WHOLE30

→ GRAIN-FREE

Total time: 35 MINUTES

EASY SKILLET CAULIFLOWER RICE JAMBALAYA *with* CHICKEN *and* SAUSAGE

- 2 tablespoons ghee
- 12 ounces fully cooked andouille or kielbasa sausage, sliced (I use no-sugar-added Wellshire Farm brand)
- ½ pound boneless, skinless chicken thighs, trimmed and cut into ½-inch cubes
- 1 medium green bell pepper, seeded and finely diced (¾ cup)
- ½ cup finely diced white onion (¼ medium)
- ¼ cup finely diced celery (1 stalk)
- 2 garlic cloves, minced
- 2 bay leaves
- ½ teaspoon cayenne pepper
- ½ teaspoon dried oregano
- ½ teaspoon dried thyme
- 1 (14.5-ounce) can diced tomatoes, drained
- ½ cup low-sodium chicken broth
- 4 cups riced cauliflower

Cauliflower rice gets a bad rap for being boring but it actually can be special. I've found that the best way to prepare it is to throw it in a skillet with fabulous flavors and spices. And when I think of what kind of dish has all that and more, it's hands-down jambalaya. Jambalaya is a dish from Louisiana consisting mainly of meat and vegetables mixed with rice. What makes it so dang good is the beautiful collection of spices added. It's a fantastic low-carb rendition that I hope you Cajun food lovers—and cauliflower rice skeptics—are going to love.

In a large skillet, melt the ghee over medium-high heat. Add the sausage and cubed chicken and cook, stirring, until the chicken is cooked through and browned on the edges, 5 to 8 minutes. Add the bell pepper, onion, and celery and cook, stirring often and scraping the bottom of the pan, until the vegetables are just tender, about 5 more minutes.

Add the garlic, bay leaves, cayenne pepper, oregano, and thyme and cook, stirring, until the garlic is tender and fragrant, about 2 minutes. Stir in the drained diced tomatoes and chicken broth and increase heat to high. Cook, stirring, until the sauce reduces by half, about 3 minutes. Reduce the heat to a simmer and add the cauliflower rice. Cook, stirring, until the rice is tender but not soggy, 3 to 4 minutes.

Taste and season with salt and pepper, if desired. Remove the bay leaves and serve.

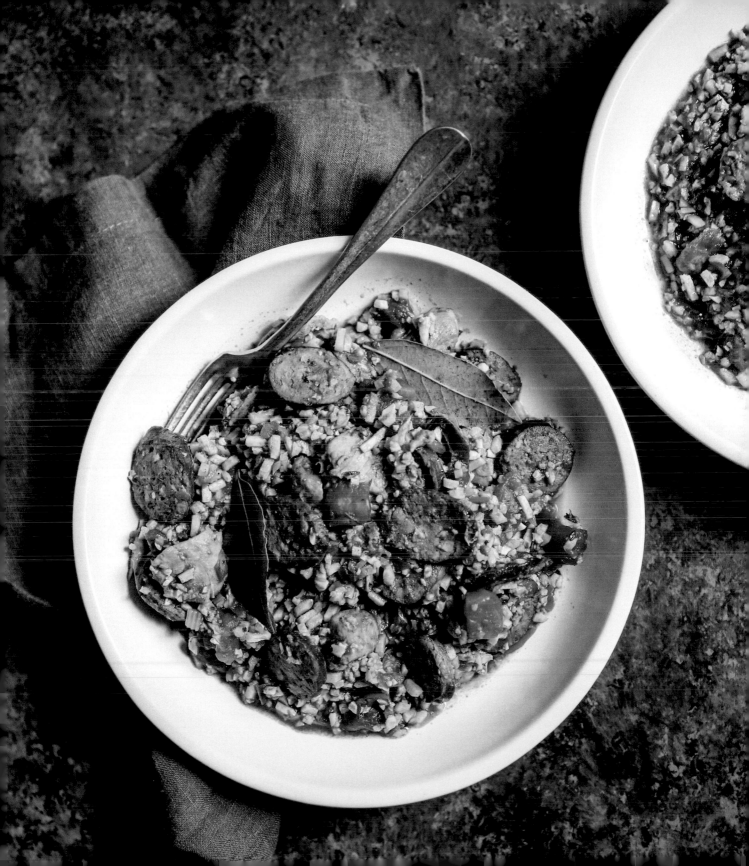

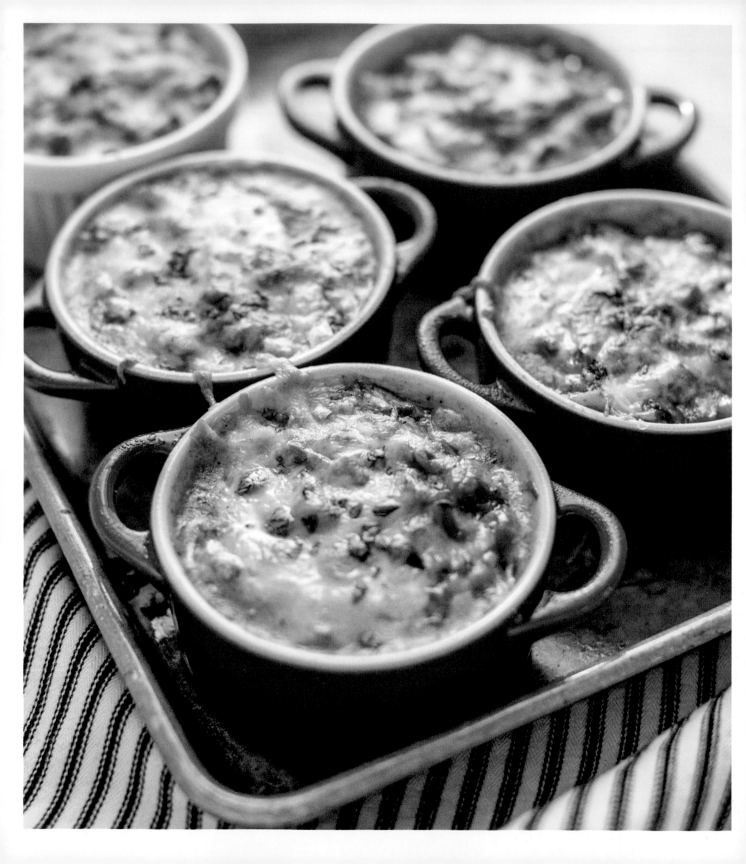

MINI KING RANCH CASSEROLES

SERVES 5

→ GLUTEN-FREE

Total time: 45 MINUTES

King Ranch, one of the largest and most historical ranches in the world, is located in Texas. Many things are named after the epic ranch, from lavish car interiors to furniture, and . . . well, creamy casseroles. The King Ranch Casserole is definitely something I grew up on living in Texas and to be honest, it was my personal favorite of all the casseroles. Typically, the ladies in town made it by combining cans of creamy soups and layering in tortillas, chicken, and chiles. This version scratches the same itch, but in a much cleaner way. And the best part? I serve it in individual ramekins so that everyone can have their own browned and bubbly casserole.

Preheat the oven to 375°F and lightly spray 5 (8-ounce) ramekins or cocottes with cooking spray.

MAKE THE SAUCE Heat a small saucepan over medium heat and melt ghee. Add the arrowroot, chili powder, garlic powder, salt, pepper, and cumin and whisk to combine. Cook, stirring, until the spices are toasted, about 2 minutes. While whisking, slowly pour in the broth and cook, stirring, until the sauce has thickened, 2 to 3 minutes. Remove from the heat and stir in the diced tomatoes and green chiles along with all the can juices. Set aside.

TO ASSEMBLE Fill the bottom of the ramekins with half of the sliced tortillas. Layer over them half of the chicken, bell pepper, and jalapeño. Pour ¼ cup of the sauce into each of the ramekins, then sprinkle with 1 cup of the cheese. Repeat by layering the remaining tortillas, chicken, bell pepper, jalapeño, and cheese, and top off with the remaining sauce.

Place the ramekins on a large baking sheet and transfer to the oven. Bake, uncovered, until the cheese is bubbly and lightly browned, 18 to 20 minutes. Let the casseroles cool for 8 to 10 minutes before sprinkling with the cilantro and serving warm.

FOR THE SAUCE

- 2 tablespoons ghee
- 2 tablespoons arrowroot starch
- ½ teaspoon chili powder
- ½ teaspoon garlic powder
- 1½ teaspoons kosher salt
- ¼ teaspoon freshly ground black pepper
- ¼ teaspoon ground cumin
- 1½ cups low-sodium chicken broth
- 1 (10-ounce) can diced tomatoes and green chiles (such as RO*TEL)

TO ASSEMBLE

- 5 gluten-free corn tortillas, halved and sliced into ½-inch slices
- 3 cups diced chicken (rotisserie or see page 279)
- ½ medium red bell pepper, seeded and finely diced (½ cup)
- ½ large jalapeño, seeded and finely diced (2 tablespoons)
- 2 cups shredded mild cheddar and Monterey jack cheese blend
- 1 tablespoon finely chopped fresh cilantro leaves

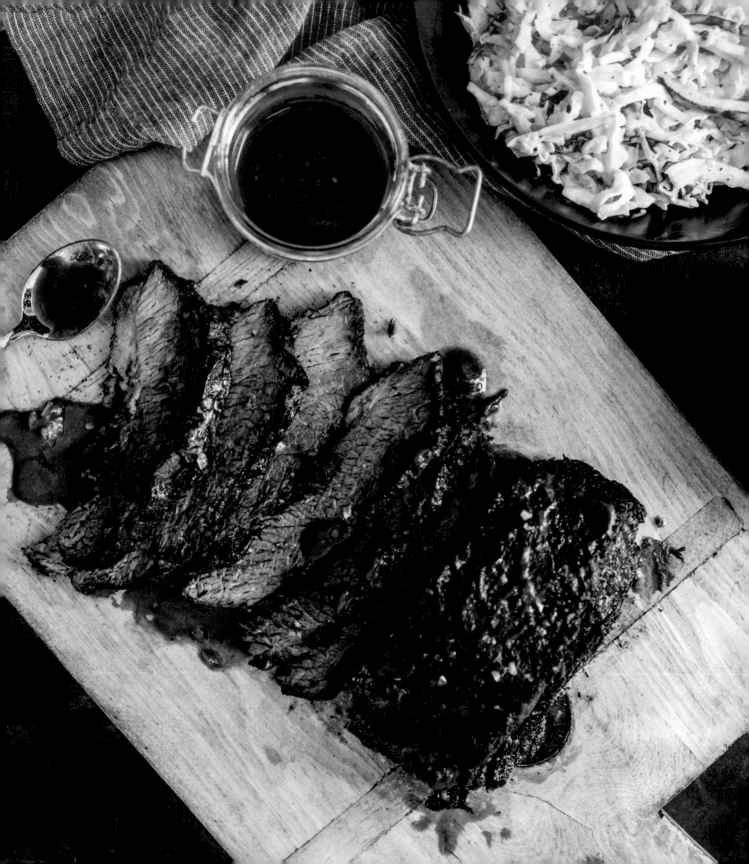

SLOW-COOKER BBQ BEEF BRISKET *with* QUICK-*and*-EASY COLESLAW

SERVES 6

→ GLUTEN-FREE
→ DAIRY-FREE
→ PALEO
→ WHOLE30
→ GRAIN-FREE

Total time: 8 HOURS, 30 MINUTES

Tender, juicy, flavorful slow-cooker beef brisket smothered in a homemade barbecue sauce . . . this is what dreams are made of! What's especially dreamy is how quick and easy this recipe is to prepare when you let your slow cooker work its magic. This brisket is great served alone with the coleslaw, or if you're feeling like treating yourself, serve it up in some buns!

MAKE THE SAUCE In a bowl, combine all the BBQ sauce ingredients and mix until well combined.

MAKE THE BRISKET Generously season the brisket all over with the salt, black pepper, smoked paprika, and cumin. Rub it into the meat with your hands.

In a large skillet, heat the oil over high heat and, when shimmering, sear brisket on all sides until a deep brown crust has formed, about 4 minutes per side.

Transfer the browned brisket into a slow cooker. Pour ½ of the BBQ sauce mixture on top. Reserve the remaining BBQ sauce in the fridge for later use. Cover and cook the brisket on low for 8 hours.

When cook time is complete, transfer the brisket onto a cutting board (reserving the juices in the slow cooker) and let rest for 10 minutes before slicing.

{ continued }

FOR THE WHOLE30 BBQ SAUCE

- ½ cup tomato sauce, no salt added
- 3 tablespoons balsamic vinegar
- 2 cloves garlic, minced
- 1 tablespoon yellow mustard
- 1 tablespoon Louisiana-style hot sauce (I like Crystal brand)
- ½ teaspoon smoked paprika

FOR THE BRISKET

- 3 pounds flat-cut brisket
- 1 tablespoon kosher salt
- 1 teaspoon freshly ground black pepper
- 1½ teaspoons smoked paprika
- 1 teaspoon ground cumin
- 2 tablespoons extra virgin olive oil
- Quick-and-Easy Coleslaw (recipe follows)

Meanwhile, transfer 2 cups of the reserved cooking liquid from the slow cooker to a small saucepan and bring to a boil over high heat. Once boiling, reduce the heat to a rapid simmer and simmer, stirring occasionally, until the liquid has reduced by half, 12 to 15 minutes.

Slice the brisket and spread across a serving platter. Pour the reduced cooking liquid over the cooked, sliced brisket.

Serve with Quick-and-Easy Coleslaw and top with extra BBQ sauce, if desired.

QUICK-AND-EASY COLESLAW

TOTAL TIME: 5 minutes

- 1 (12-ounce) bag coleslaw mix
- ½ cup homemade mayo (page 281)
- 1 teaspoon Dijon mustard
- 2 cloves garlic, minced
- 2 tablespoons white vinegar
- 1 teaspoon kosher salt
- ½ teaspoon freshly ground black pepper

Combine all ingredients in a bowl and toss until well combined. Refrigerate until ready to serve and serve within at least 2 hours!

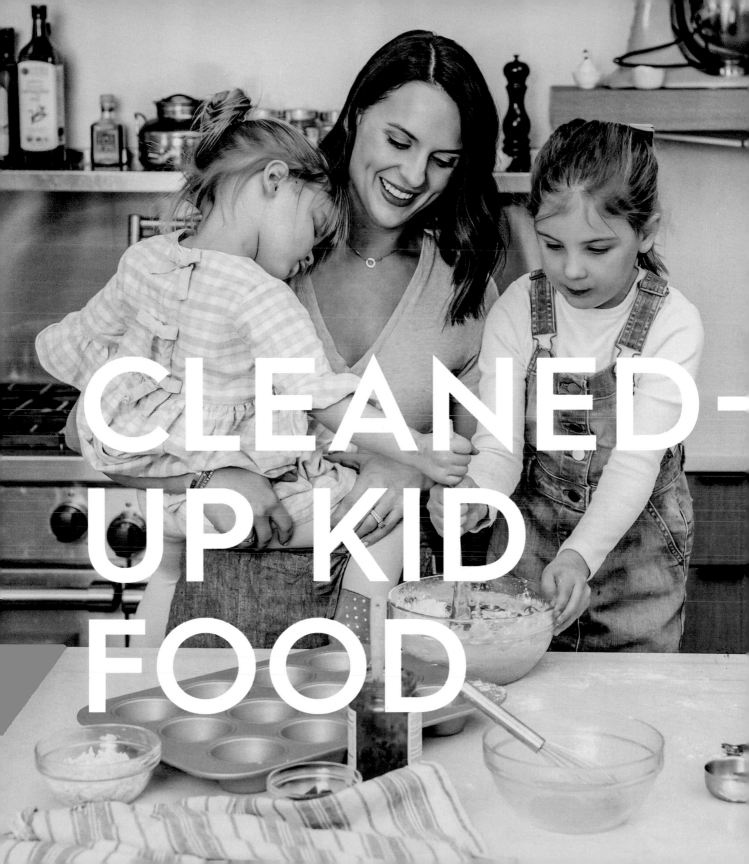

CLEANED-UP KID FOOD

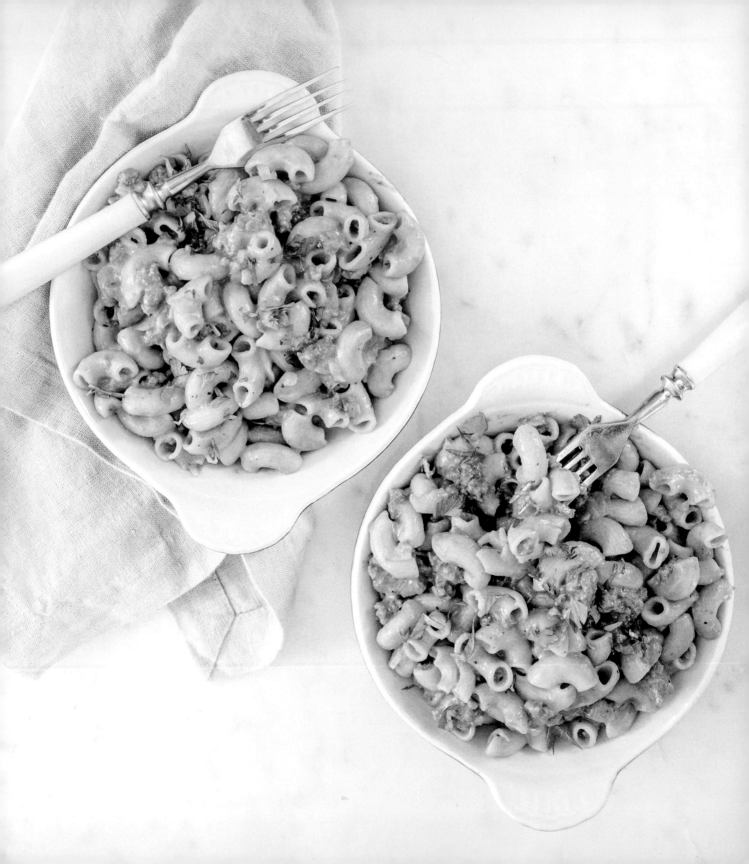

ONE-POT HAMBURGER HELPER

SERVES 4

→ GLUTEN-FREE

→ DAIRY-FREE IF MODIFIED

Total time: 25 MINUTES

Cue all of the nostalgic '90s feelings . . . because Hamburger Helper is making a comeback! I used to love really busy nights when my mom had zero time to cook and would make this just-add-meat classic because, let's be honest, that stuff was freaking good. Although the kid in me wants to make a box every once in a while, the adult in me knows way too much about processed food to go there. That's why I have created my own cleaned-up version that's a total crowd pleaser and honestly? Just as easy as the boxed version. With one pot and 30 minutes, you'll have a meal on the table that the whole family will devour.

In a large, high-sided skillet or pot, heat the oil over medium-high heat. Add the beef, onion, salt, pepper, garlic powder, and paprika and cook, breaking up the beef with the back of a spoon, until the meat is browned and no longer pink, 5 to 7 minutes.

Add the tomato paste and stir until it is well combined with the beef. Stir in the pasta, broth, and milk. Bring the mixture to a boil and reduce to a simmer. Cook, stirring often, until the pasta is tender, 10 to 13 minutes.

Fold in the cheese, if using. Taste and adjust the seasoning with more salt and pepper, if desired. Sprinkle with parsley and serve hot.

- 2 tablespoons extra virgin olive oil
- 1 pound ground beef, 90 percent lean
- ½ medium onion, finely diced (1 cup)
- 1 teaspoon kosher salt
- ½ teaspoon freshly ground black pepper
- ½ teaspoon garlic powder
- ½ teaspoon paprika
- 1 tablespoon tomato paste
- 12 ounces uncooked gluten-free elbow pasta (I use Jovial brand)
- 2 cups low-sodium beef broth
- 2 cups whole milk (use unsweetened almond milk for dairy-free)
- 1 cup shredded mild cheddar cheese (omit for dairy-free)
- ¼ cup chopped fresh flat-leaf parsley leaves

from MY KITCHEN to YOURS

Heat leftovers over medium heat and add ¼ cup beef broth to rehydrate the noodles until tender and creamy again.

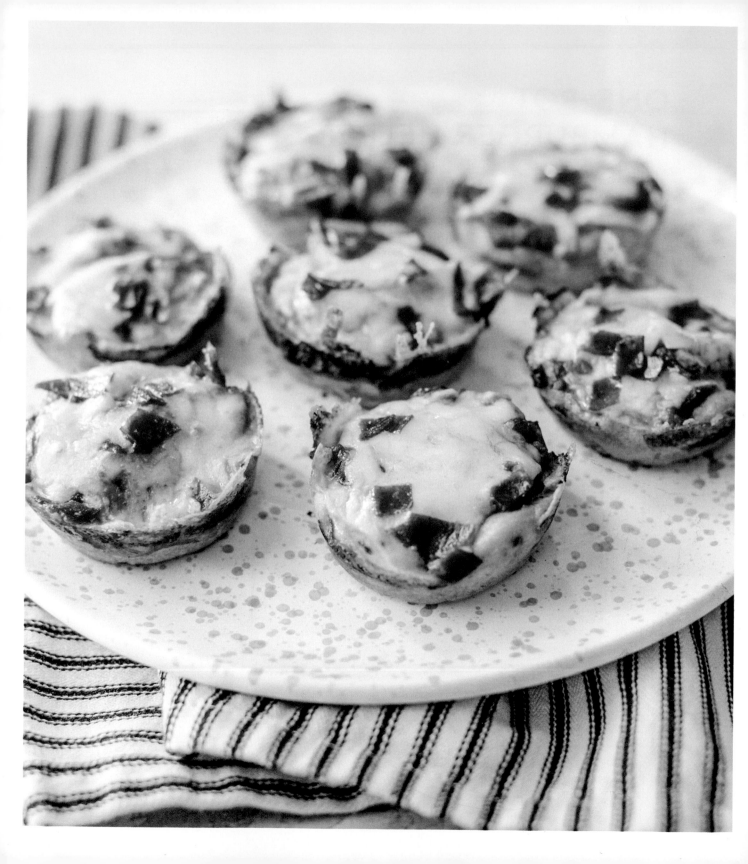

GRAIN-FREE PIZZA BITES

MAKES 12 BITES

→ GLUTEN-FREE

→ GRAIN-FREE

Total time: 30 MINUTES

Apparently the '90s loved pizza. We had Bagel Bites, Hot Pockets, Pizza Rolls, pizza Lunchables . . . even pizza-flavored chips! Don't get me wrong, I am all for it, but just knowing that our childhood favorites had nearly no *real, clean* ingredients in them makes me cringe a bit. But, that will never stop me from finding a way for my own kiddos to enjoy my childhood favorites. And, wow, do my kiddos LOVE these mini pizza bites. It's like all of our '90s pizza-flavored dreams bundled up into one, small, clean-eating bite! So bake up some of these for you and your kiddos and tell them about how cool you were in the '90s. When they take a bite of these, they might just believe you!

FOR THE CRUST

- 1 cup cassava flour
- ¼ cup arrowroot starch
- 1 teaspoon kosher salt
- 1 teaspoon Italian seasoning
- 2 large eggs
- ¼ cup extra virgin olive oil

FOR THE TOPPING

- ½ cup pizza sauce or jarred marinara (I use Rao's Homemade brand)
- ¼ cup shredded Italian cheese blend (plain shredded mozzarella or provolone works, too)
- 8 pepperoni slices, diced small

Preheat the oven to 425°F and lightly grease a 12-cup muffin tin with nonstick cooking spray.

MAKE THE CRUST In a mixing bowl, combine the cassava, arrowroot, salt, and Italian seasoning. Stir to combine.

In a separate bowl, combine eggs, olive oil, and ½ cup cold water. Whisk until frothy.

Pour egg mixture over the dry ingredients and, using a rubber spatula, stir to combine. Let sit for 5 minutes to allow the dough to firm up a bit.

Drop about 1 tablespoon of the dough into each greased muffin cup. With wet fingertips, gently press down the dough until it is in an even layer. Transfer to the oven and bake until the dough is firm, about 10 minutes.

Remove dough from oven and top each pizza bite with 1 teaspoon pizza sauce, a sprinkle of cheese, and diced pepperoni. Place back in the oven and bake until the cheese is melted and bubbly, about 5 more minutes.

Remove from oven and let cool in the muffin tin so that the cheese firms up a bit and the bites stay together, about 5 more minutes.

SERVES 4

→ GLUTEN-FREE

→ DAIRY-FREE

→ PALEO

→ WHOLE30

→ GRAIN-FREE

Total time: 45 MINUTES
BUT DON'T FORGET TO LET
YOUR CHICKEN MARINATE
FIRST!

THE BEST GRAIN-FREE CHICKEN NUGGETS

1½ pounds boneless, skinless breasts

½ cup dill pickle juice

2 large eggs

½ cup tapioca starch

½ cup almond flour

1 teaspoon garlic powder

1 teaspoon onion powder

1 teaspoon sweet paprika

1½ teaspoons kosher salt

1 teaspoon freshly ground black pepper

½ cup avocado oil

Dipping sauce of your choice, for serving

If I had a cleaned-up kids' food section of this book without some sort of chicken finger or nugget in it, what kind of mom/cookbook author would I be? Is there anything more kid-approved than a chicken nugget?

My kids favorite "restaurant" just so happens to be the drive-through with the best chicken nuggets ever . . . yeah, you know which one I am referring to, right? I can't lie to you either, it's a guilty pleasure for me as well. I've re-created those nuggets (sans junk) in my own kitchen, and oh-my-good-heavens they are freaking good. Definitely the best paleo nugget I've ever tasted. The trick? Brine your nuggets in pickle juice. It makes them much more tender and oh-so-flavorful!

Lay the chicken breasts in a single layer across a cutting board and cover with plastic wrap or parchment paper. Using a meat mallet or the bottom of a skillet, pound the breasts until they are an even ¼-inch thickness. Remove and discard the plastic wrap, then cut the chicken into 2-inch pieces.

Place the chicken in a bowl with the pickle juice, and toss to coat evenly. Cover and refrigerate to allow the chicken to brine in the pickle juice for at least 2 hours (and up to all day).

When chicken has finished brining, strain off the excess pickle juice.

Set up an assembly line for dredging your chicken: In a shallow bowl, whisk together the eggs and 1 tablespoon water until frothy. In a separate shallow bowl, combine the tapioca starch, almond

{ continued }

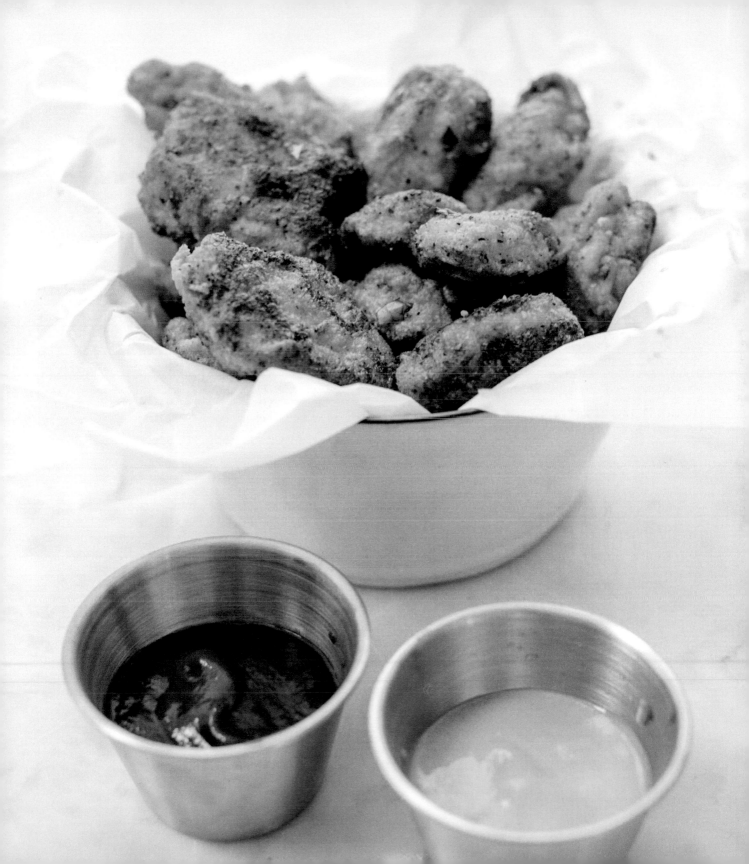

flour, garlic powder, onion powder, paprika, salt, and black pepper. Using a fork, stir to combine and break up any clumps.

Individually dip each chicken piece in the egg, letting excess drip off, then roll in the flour mixture to coat. Set aside on a clean plate and continue until all the chicken is coated. To make your dredging process cleaner, I like to designate one hand to dip the chicken into the egg mixture, then the other for the rolling in the flour mixture.

In a Dutch oven, heat the avocado oil over medium heat. When hot, working in batches, fry the chicken until the crust is golden brown and the meat is cooked through, about 3 minutes on the first side, and 1 to 2 minutes on the second. Once cooked, transfer chicken to a paper towel–lined plate and continue until all the chicken is cooked through and crispy.

Serve with your favorite dipping sauce.

AIR FRYER METHOD

After you have set up your assembly line, preheat your air fryer to 400°F for 8 minutes. In two separate batches, dredge the chicken and place in the air fryer basket, being careful not to overcrowd the basket so that the chicken has plenty of room to crisp up all around. Spray the tops generously with avocado oil spray and cook for 5 minutes. Pull the basket out, carefully flip the nuggets over, and spray the other side with avocado oil spray. Continue to cook for 4 more minutes, or until the chicken is crispy all over and cooked through. Remove from the air fryer and transfer the cooked nuggets to a paper towel-lined plate and continue until all of the chicken is cooked.

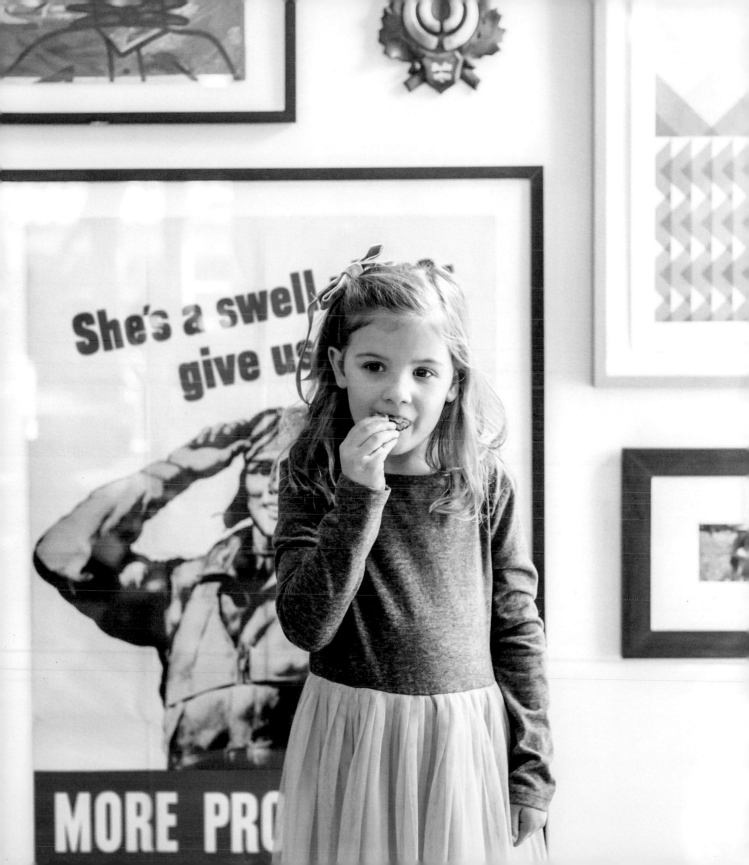

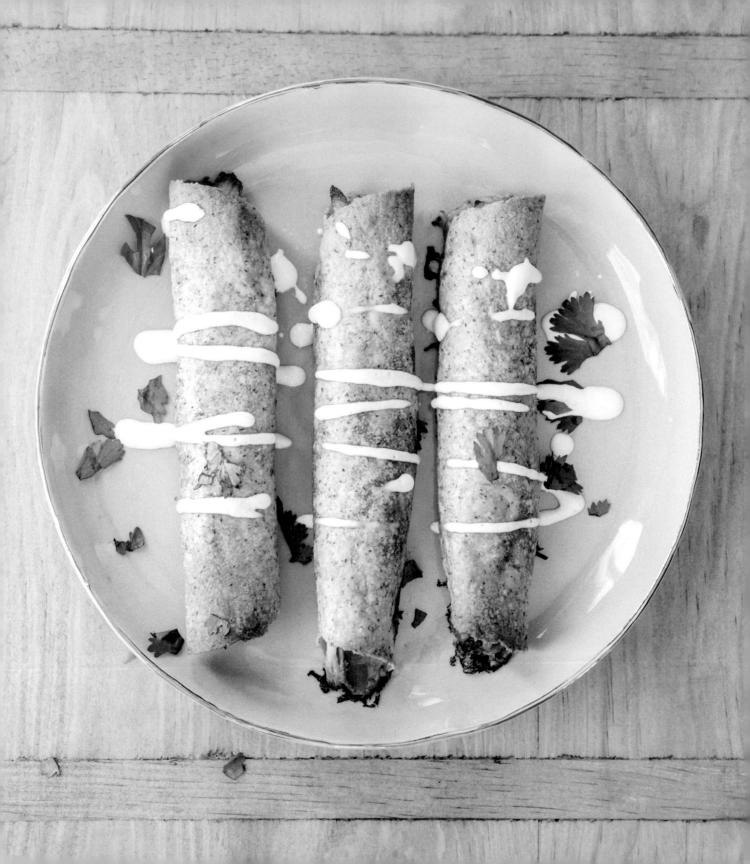

SOUR CREAM CHICKEN TAQUITOS

SERVES 4

→ GLUTEN-FREE

→ GRAIN-FREE

Total time: 30 MINUTES

Growing up, one of my favorite frozen foods to heat up for an after-school snack was taquitos. Now I love making them because they're easy to throw together and perfect for on-the-go meals. This version is cleaner than the store-bought original (though no less delicious), and is a fixture in our house because the taquitos can be frozen and make for great school lunches reheated.

1½ cups shredded chicken (rotisserie or see page 279)

1 cup roughly chopped baby spinach

1 (4-ounce) can mild green chiles, undrained

½ cup sour cream

½ cup shredded mild cheddar cheese

½ teaspoon kosher salt

¼ teaspoon freshly ground black pepper

Avocado oil, for cooking the tortillas

8 (8-inch) gluten-free corn tortillas or grain-free tortillas (I use Siete brand)

Preheat the oven to 400°F. Line a large baking sheet with parchment paper and set aside.

In a large bowl, combine the shredded chicken, spinach, chiles, sour cream, shredded cheese, salt, and pepper. Stir until well combined.

In a small, nonstick skillet, heat about 1 teaspoon of the avocado oil over medium-high heat. Quickly fry 1 tortilla at a time until flexible and easy to roll, about 30 seconds per side. Immediately fill the tortilla with about 2 tablespoons of the chicken mixture and gently roll up. Place seam-side down on the prepared baking sheet. Repeat with the remaining tortillas, adding more oil to the skillet as needed.

Transfer the baking sheet to the oven and bake until the taquitos are crispy and brown on the edges, about 20 minutes. Let cool for 10 minutes before serving, or cool completely to freeze.

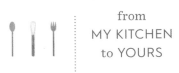

from
MY KITCHEN
to YOURS

These are perfect for freezing and reheating! Allow taquitos to cool to room temperature, then place in a single layer in a freezer bag and lay them flat in your freezer. To reheat, microwave for 2 to 4 minutes, or pop in the oven at 450°F for about 10 minutes.

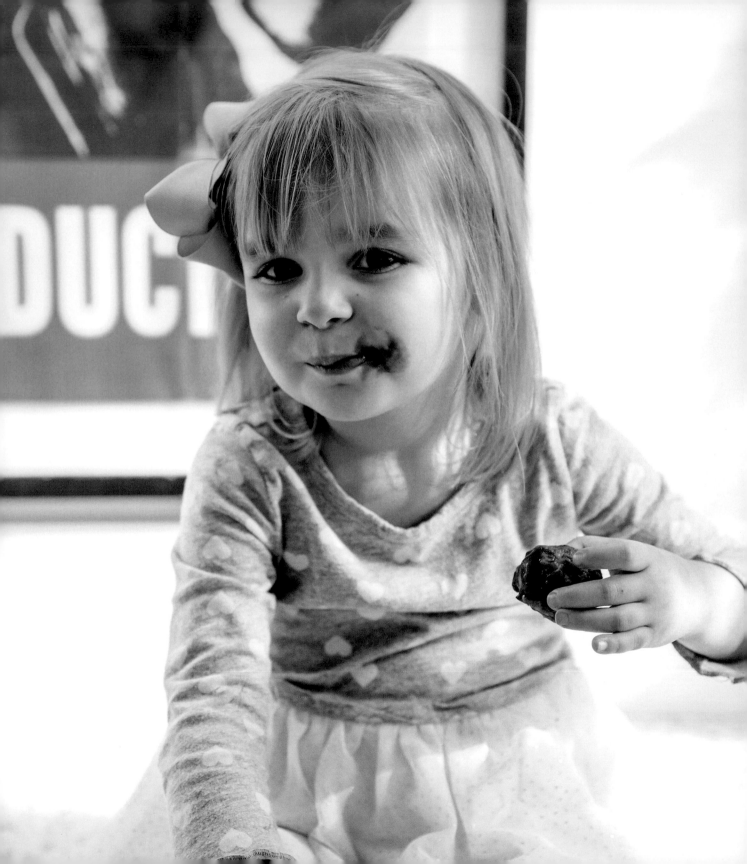

CHEESEBURGER MEATBALLS

SERVES 4

→ GLUTEN-FREE

→ GRAIN-FREE

Total time: 30 MINUTES

Adults or kids, there aren't many folks who don't love a good ole cheeseburger. To make life easier on the go, I came up with these cheeseburger-inspired meatballs that have all the makings of a classic cheeseburger, just packed into a portable meatball. I love making these at the beginning of the week to pop into lunch boxes or to serve as an after-school snack.

Preheat the oven to 400°F. Line a baking sheet with parchment paper and set aside.

In a large bowl, combine the beef, cheese, almond flour, egg, relish, ketchup, mustard, salt, garlic powder, onion powder, and pepper. Using your hands, mix until well combined. Form the meat mixture into twelve 1½ inch balls (or use a generous tablespoon scoop). Place the meatballs on the prepared baking sheet. Bake until cooked through, about 15 minutes. Enjoy immediately or let cool completely before storing in the fridge for up to 5 days.

1 pound ground beef, 90 percent lean

1 cup shredded mild cheddar cheese

¼ cup almond flour

1 large egg

2 tablespoons dill relish

1 tablespoon ketchup (I use unsweetened Primal Kitchen brand)

1 teaspoon Dijon mustard

1 teaspoon kosher salt

½ teaspoon garlic powder

½ teaspoon onion powder

½ teaspoon freshly ground black pepper

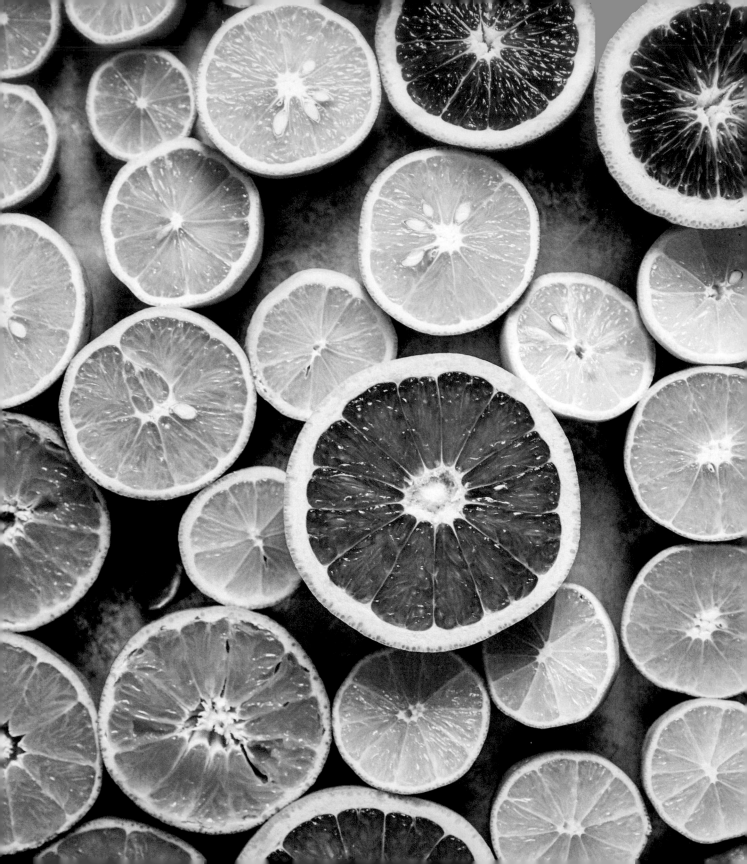

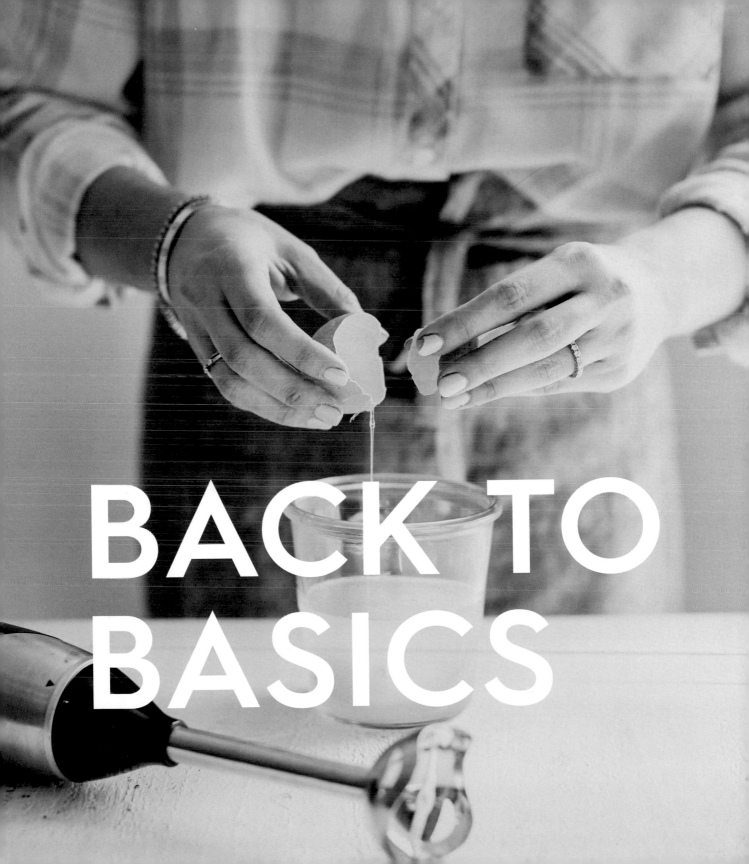

BACK TO BASICS

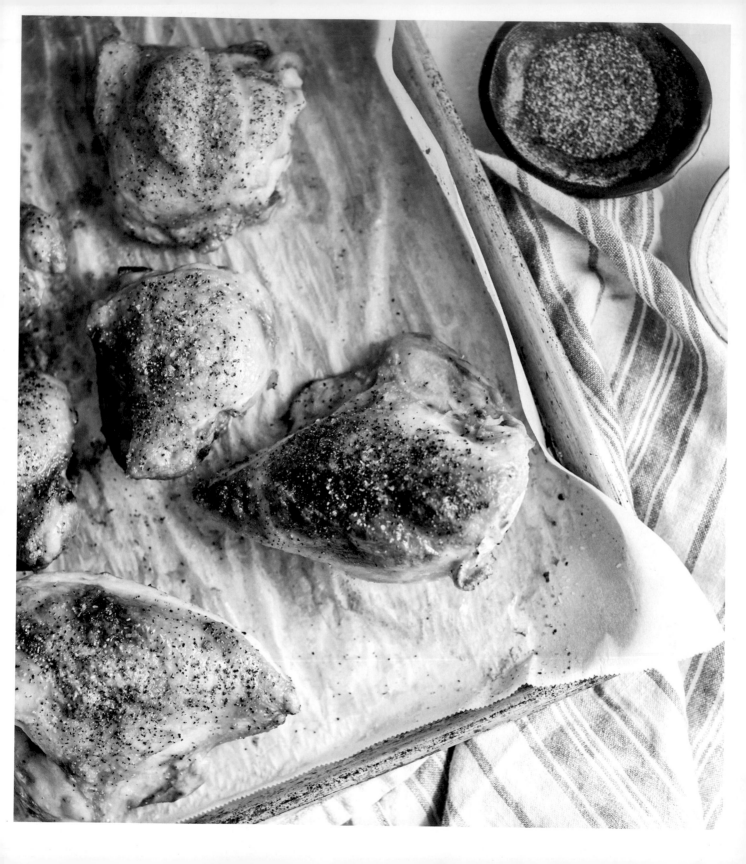

SIMPLE ROASTED CHICKEN

MAKES ABOUT 6 CUPS
SHREDDED CHICKEN

→ GLUTEN-FREE

→ DAIRY-FREE

→ PALEO

→ WHOLE30

→ GRAIN-FREE

Total time: 1 HOUR

Everyone needs a good roasted chicken recipe to use in recipes, and this is mine. I sometimes eat this chicken as it is alongside roasted veggies, but for the most part, I shred it up to use in soups, salads, chicken salads . . . or really anything that calls for shredded chicken. I like to make a batch of this at the beginning of the week for meal prep so that I can use it as needed in recipes. Throughout this book you'll see me call for shredded chicken, and I will be sending you right back to this page to make it this way! You can also use store-bought rotisserie chicken in those recipes if you are in a hurry.

4 bone-in, skin-on chicken breasts (about 2½ pounds)

4 bone-in, skin-on chicken thighs (about 1½ pounds)

2 tablespoons extra virgin olive oil

2 teaspoons kosher salt

1 teaspoon freshly ground pepper black pepper

Preheat the oven to 375°F. Cover a large baking sheet with parchment paper.

Place the chicken breasts and thighs on top of the parchment paper and drizzle with the olive oil. Rub the olive oil all over the chicken pieces to coat evenly. Season the tops with the salt and pepper.

Place the baking sheet in the preheated oven and bake until the thighs are cooked through, about 35 minutes.

Keep the oven on and, using tongs, carefully transfer the chicken thighs to a large cutting board to let rest. Return the baking sheet with the breasts back to the oven and continue to cook for about 10 more minutes, or until the meat is no longer pink and the juices run clear.

Allow all of the chicken to rest for about 10 minutes before eating it as-is or, to use in recipes, let cool enough to handle with your hands. Peel and discard the skin and, using your hands, pull/shred the chicken into bite-size pieces.

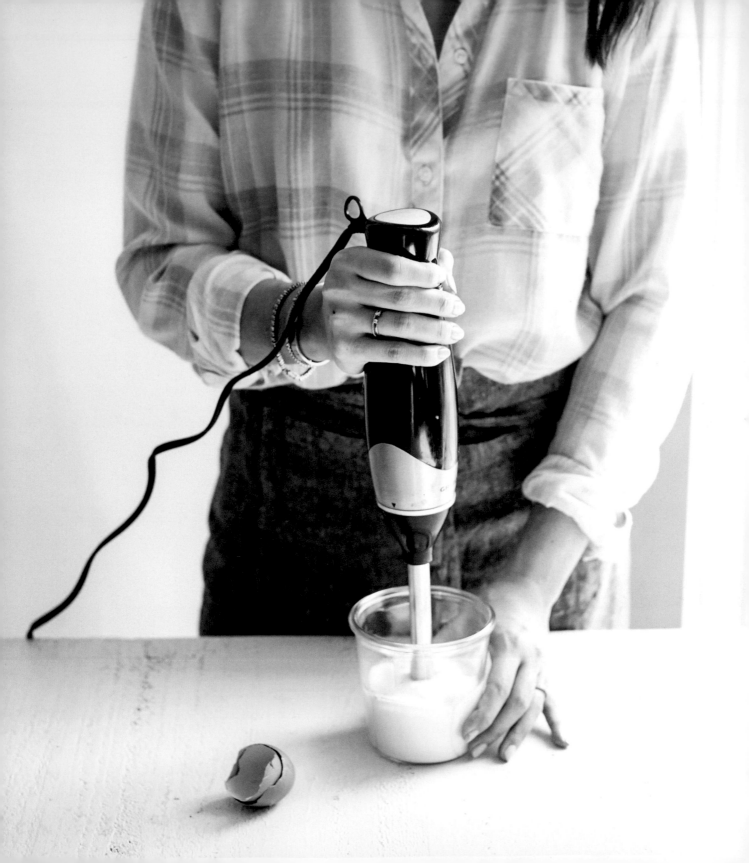

ONE-MINUTE IMMERSION BLENDER MAYO BASE

MAKES 1 CUP

→ GLUTEN-FREE

→ DAIRY-FREE

→ PALEO

→ WHOLE30

→ GRAIN-FREE

Total time: 1 MINUTES

The first time I completed a Whole30 challenge, I had never used or made homemade mayo. What a disservice I was doing to myself! You may think, what on earth could I use mayo for that would make such a difference? A ton of things! In this book, you'll see that I use this simple mayo base to create fantastic salad dressings, sauces, and dips to elevate everyday food. It takes about 1 minute to make and the possibilities are truly endless.

Pour the oil into a wide-mouth glass jar with an opening a little bit wider than the head of your immersion blender. Crack the egg into the oil and let settle into the bottom of the jar.

Place the immersion blender into the jar and position the blade directly over the egg yolk. Turn the immersion blender on low and hold in place, while the blender is running, until the bottom of the jar starts to turn into a creamy emulsion, about 10 seconds. Once you see that creamy emulsion at the bottom, start lifting the blender up a bit and pressing it back down, essentially emulsifying the mixture above the mayo at the bottom, bit by bit, until you reach the top and the entire jar is emulsified. Use as-is in the recipes throughout this book.

OPTIONAL You can turn it into actual mayo by blending in the optional ingredients.

1 cup avocado oil or other light-flavored oil

1 large egg

OPTIONAL

1 clove minced garlic

1 teaspoon fresh lemon juice

2 teaspoons mustard powder

Kosher salt to taste

SERVES 4

→ GLUTEN-FREE

→ DAIRY-FREE

→ PALEO

→ WHOLE30

→ GRAIN-FREE

Total time: 10 MINUTES

PREPARED CAULIFLOWER RICE

1 large head cauliflower, cut into small pieces

1 tablespoon extra virgin olive oil

Kosher salt

Freshly ground black pepper

While eating a mostly grain-free, gluten-free diet, cauliflower has become one of the most versatile vegetables and I love experimenting with it. One of my favorite things to do is to turn it into "rice" and use as a substitute in dishes where there would normally be a starch. Plus, it's a great way to squeeze more servings of veggies into your diet.

Place the cauliflower pieces in a food processor (depending on the size of your food processor, you will likely need to do this in 2 batches). Pulse the food processor until the cauliflower is the texture of rice, or "riced."

Heat the oil in a large skillet over medium-high heat. When shimmering, add the riced cauliflower and cook, stirring, until heated through, 3 to 5 minutes. Don't overcook the cauliflower rice, or it tends to get mushy. Season with salt and pepper to taste and serve as desired.

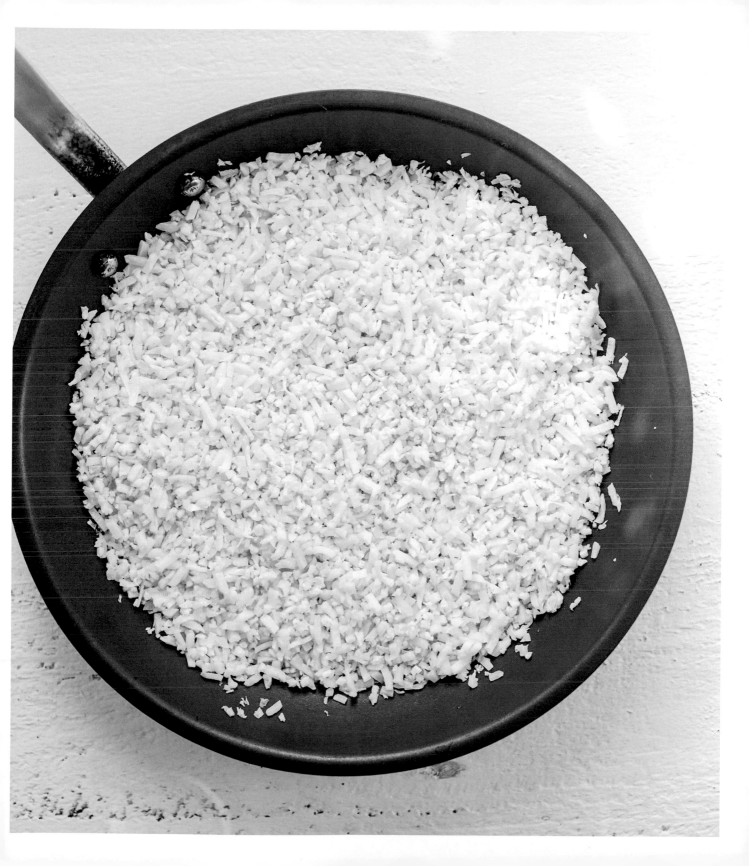

SERVES 4

→ GLUTEN-FREE

→ DAIRY-FREE

→ PALEO

→ WHOLE30

→ GRAIN-FREE

Total time: 40 MINUTES
(OR 8 MINUTES USING AN
INSTANT POT)

1 medium-size spaghetti squash
  (2 to 3 pounds)

2 tablespoons extra virgin
  olive oil

1 teaspoon kosher salt

ROASTED SPAGHETTI SQUASH

Spaghetti squash is one of those magical vegetables that still blows my mind. No spiralizers or special gadgets required, this vegetable (when cooked correctly) transforms into tender tangles of spaghetti! My favorite way to cook spaghetti squash is to roast in the oven, as I prefer its roasted flavor; however, it takes 30 to 40 minutes. If I am in a hurry to get dinner on the table, I will pop my spaghetti squash in my Instant Pot, and in a magical 8 minutes, the spaghetti squash is ready to be served! Throughout this book, you'll see me mention that you can serve a lot of my dishes over spaghetti squash, and here is how I make it.

Preheat the oven to 400°F and line a baking sheet with parchment paper.

Using a sharp knife, first trim off a small slice from each end of the spaghetti squash and discard. Next, cut the spaghetti squash in half crosswise. Using a sharp spoon (I use an ice cream scoop), scoop out the seeds and stringy bits from the center of each cavity and discard.

Place the squash, cavity-side up, on the prepared baking sheet and brush the inside all over with the olive oil. Sprinkle with salt and roast until fork-tender, 30 to 35 minutes.

Remove the squash from oven and allow to cool enough to handle. Using a fork, gently scrape out the strands that resemble spaghetti. Serve as desired.

{ continued }

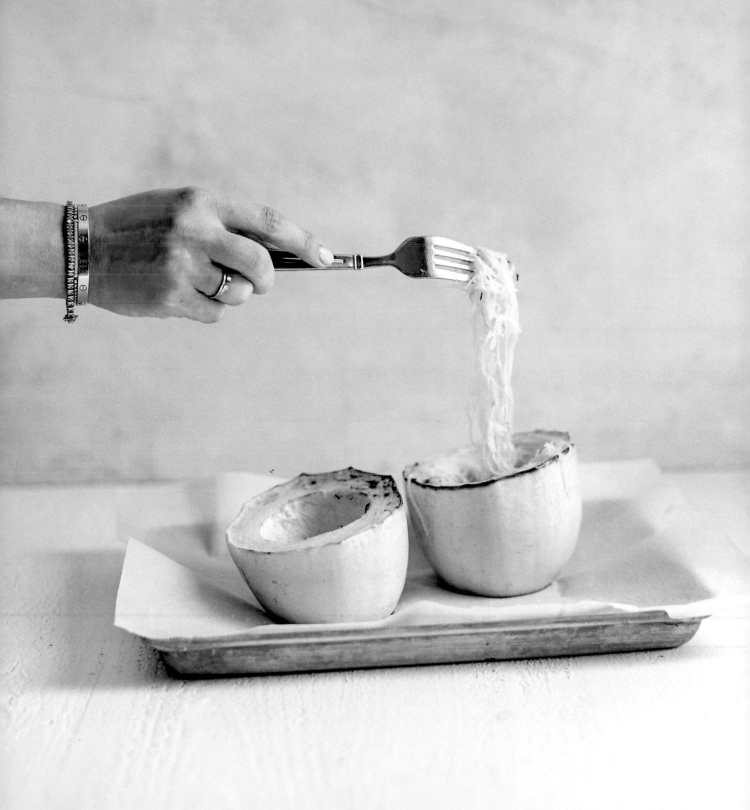

INSTANT POT METHOD

Total time: 8 minutes

1 medium-size spaghetti squash (2 to 3 pounds)

Using a sharp knife, first trim off a small slice from each end of the spaghetti squash and discard.

Next, cut the spaghetti squash in half crosswise. Using a sharp spoon (I use an ice cream scoop) scoop out the seeds and stringy bits from the center of each cavity and discard.

Place the steamer insert into your Instant Pot and add 1 cup of water. Place the squash halves on top of the steamer insert, cut side up.

Close the lid on the Instant Pot and make sure the valve is sealed. Cook under high pressure for 8 minutes. When the cook time is complete, carefully turn the valve to rapidly release the pressure.

When the pressure has released, remove the lid from the pot. When cool enough to handle, tip the squash halves to pour out any collected liquid. Transfer cooked squash to a cutting board or plate and gently scrape out the strands that resemble spaghetti. Serve as desired.

INDEX

NOTE: Page references in *italics* refer to photos of recipes.

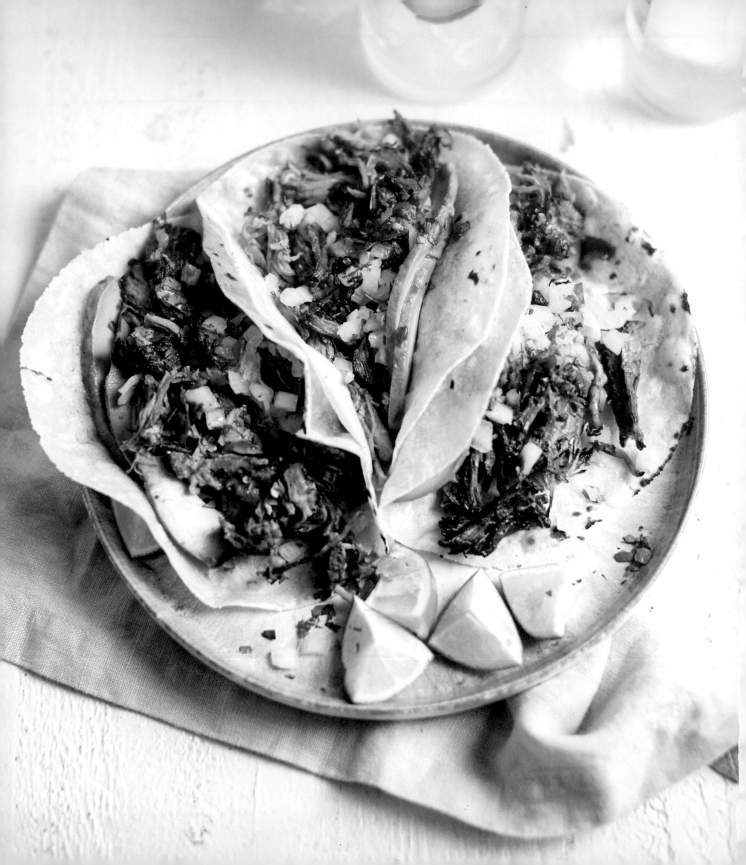

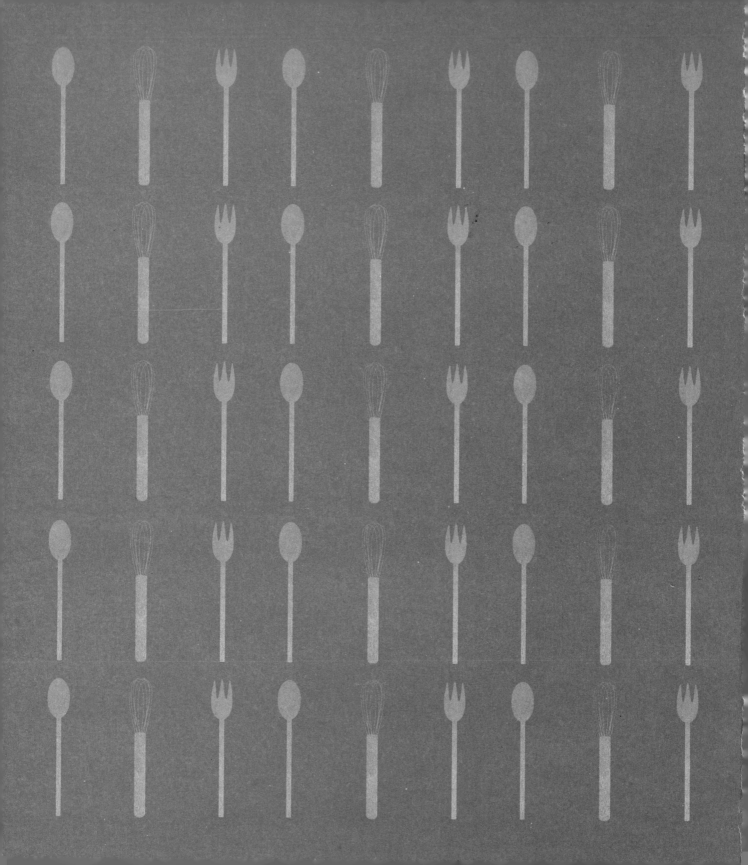